AF761854

Major Pandemics

Iain K Crombie

Major Pandemics

Where They Come from, Why They Spread, and When They End

palgrave
macmillan

Iain K Crombie
Division of Population Health and Genomics
Dundee University
Dundee, UK

ISBN 978-981-95-2080-0 ISBN 978-981-95-2081-7 (eBook)
https://doi.org/10.1007/978-981-95-2081-7

© The Editor(s) (if applicable) and The Author(s), under exclusive license to Springer Nature Singapore Pte Ltd. 2025

This work is subject to copyright. All rights are solely and exclusively licensed by the Publisher, whether the whole or part of the material is concerned, specifically the rights of translation, reprinting, reuse of illustrations, recitation, broadcasting, reproduction on microfilms or in any other physical way, and transmission or information storage and retrieval, electronic adaptation, computer software, or by similar or dissimilar methodology now known or hereafter developed.
The use of general descriptive names, registered names, trademarks, service marks, etc. in this publication does not imply, even in the absence of a specific statement, that such names are exempt from the relevant protective laws and regulations and therefore free for general use.
The publisher, the authors and the editors are safe to assume that the advice and information in this book are believed to be true and accurate at the date of publication. Neither the publisher nor the authors or the editors give a warranty, expressed or implied, with respect to the material contained herein or for any errors or omissions that may have been made. The publisher remains neutral with regard to jurisdictional claims in published maps and institutional affiliations.

This Palgrave Macmillan imprint is published by the registered company Springer Nature Singapore Pte Ltd.
The registered company address is: 152 Beach Road, #21-01/04 Gateway East, Singapore 189721, Singapore

If disposing of this product, please recycle the paper.

Acknowledgements

This book emerged from a career-long interest in diseases, and the free time that comes with the post of emeritus professor. I am deeply grateful to the University of Dundee for providing the facilities that enabled me to research and write this book. The computing staff who run the Help4U support system solved some technical problems, and Kayleigh McGarry of the Library sorted out all my referencing difficulties. Family and friends provided the support and encouragement that enabled me to complete the manuscript, with Helen, Neville, Liz, David and Terri providing comments on individual chapters. Thank you all.

Contents

Introduction

Hot, dry winds forever blowing,
Dead men to the grave-yards going:
Constant hearses,
Funeral verses;
Oh! what plagues—there is no knowing![1]

Infectious diseases have been a constant feature of human existence. Some are ancient. For example, the viruses that cause chickenpox, herpes and hepatitis co-evolved with our distant ancestors millions of years ago. The whooping cough bacterium, *Bordetella pertussis*, is not quite so old at about 1 million years ago. In contrast *Helicobacter pylori*, the bacterium which causes stomach ulcers, is a little more recent: it probably accompanied humans as they migrated out of Africa 40–60,000 years ago. These are all examples of what are commonly called the heirloom diseases, infections which have been around for a long time but are still causing illness today [1–5].

Possibly the oldest and certainly the strangest of the heirloom microbes are the human endogenous retroviruses. These were RNA viruses that

[1] The first verse of a poem entitled 'Pestilence' by Philip Freneau (1752–1832). Written about an outbreak of yellow fever in Philadelphia, 1793.

© The Author(s), under exclusive license to Springer Nature Singapore Pte Ltd. 2025
I. K Crombie, *Major Pandemics*, https://doi.org/10.1007/978-981-95-2081-7_1

once infected our far distant ancestors. Then about 35–40 million years ago they integrated themselves into the DNA of their hosts and since then have been transmitted genetically from parents to children. Today the remnants of these ancient viruses make up about 5–8% of human DNA. Not all of them are simply passengers; some play important roles in the regulation of the biochemistry of human cells. But others are involved in the development of diseases such as cancer, schizophrenia and multiple sclerosis [6, 7].

Currently about 1500 species of bacteria and 270 of viral species are known to cause disease in humans. These numbers are likely to be underestimates because the more that scientists investigate, the more they find new microorganisms that can invade humans. What is reassuring is that major outbreaks of illness and death are uncommon. A 2007 study estimated that only 25 of these diseases have caused widespread infection in the recent past (i.e. the last 1000 years). Since then another two diseases have been added to the list: swine flu in 2009 and the 2019 Covid pandemic. There have been other large outbreaks of disease in the more distant past, but less is known about them [1, 8–10].

Early Outbreaks of Infectious Diseases

The nature and size of ancient outbreaks of infectious diseases are not known, as little information is provided by historical records. Most likely those people who began living in towns and cities several thousand years ago had more pressing things to do than record illnesses. An early source, the Old Testament, identifies ten plagues in Egypt, although only two of them affected humans. One caused an outbreak of boils and the other killed all first-born children. The others involved the water of the river Nile turning bloody and foul, plagues of frogs, swarms of insects, severe weather events and a darkness that obscured all light [11].

One of the first large outbreaks to be described in some detail was the Plague of Athens (430–426 BCE). The cause of this plague is unknown, although many candidates have been proposed, including bubonic plague, typhoid, typhus, smallpox and measles. There is agreement that the common symptoms were red pustules on the skin, high fever, foul breath, violent coughing, severe pain, retching and diarrhoea. The combination of an unpleasant disease, and an estimated mortality rate of about 30%, led to severe social disruption. Laws and religious practices were ignored, immoral behaviour was common and many of the dead were left unburied or were cast into communal burial pits. The Plague of Athens may also have changed history. In the Peloponnesian War, the Athenians were weakened by disease and were defeated by their old rival, the Spartans. This hastened the end of the golden age of Athenian culture [12, 13].

About 400 years after the Plague of Athens, the Roman Empire suffered from a virulent disease. Named the Antonine Plague after the dynasty that was in power at the time, it wreaked havoc from 165 to 180 CE. The infection may have been brought to Italy by soldiers return ing from conquests in Mesopotamia (present-day Iraq). The symptoms included a widespread rash, diarrhoea which was initially light brown but later turned black, and a cough. Based on the writings of Galen, a Greek physician working in Rome in 165 CE, the disease may have been smallpox. It is thought to have killed somewhere between 2% and 25% of the population. (Estimates of death rates from historical documents often vary greatly) [14–16].

What Are Pandemics?

These two disease outbreaks were undoubtedly destructive but were they pandemics? Perhaps surprisingly, there is no agreed definition of the term 'pandemic'. The term comes from two Greek words: *pan* meaning all and *demos* the people, but that isn't very helpful. It raises the question of which people, where they were and what was happening to them. The World Health Organization has given some helpful descriptions of a pandemic, without ever providing a formal definition. One text simply refers to 'the worldwide spread of a new disease', and another mentions 'increased and sustained transmission in the general population'. A much more detailed one refers to a disease that has caused 'several outbreaks in at least one country, and to have spread to other countries, with consistent disease patterns indicating that serious morbidity and mortality is likely in at least one segment of the population'. This is consistent with a commonly used definition. It states that a pandemic is 'an epidemic occurring over a very wide area, crossing international boundaries, and usually affecting a large number of people' [17, 18].

Some academics are not content with the commonly used definition. They assert that pandemics must have at least one or more additional features such as being highly infectious, spreading rapidly across countries and causing severe disease. Another suggested requirement is that the people in region where the infection is spreading should have low levels of immunity to the disease. Certainly, three pandemics of the last 100 years meet all these additional criteria. Spanish flu, HIV and Covid 19 were highly infectious and spread rapidly round the world, each killing more than 5 million people. In addition, each new country they infected had low levels of immunity [17–21].

The problem is that many pandemics do not fit all these criteria. Rapid spread was not possible for some pandemics. The Black Death took about eight years to spread from its home in central Asia to arrive in Europe. Similarly, from an initial large outbreak in Italy, syphilis took two years to spread across Europe, and a few more years to spread round the world. Meeting the severity criterion is easy for diseases like smallpox, Spanish flu (influenza) and Covid-19. But should leprosy and polio be excluded because, although they are responsible for widespread illness and disability, they cause few deaths. The extent of human suffering is just as important as the number of people who died. This book adopts the straightforward definition. A pandemic is a disease that has spread across many countries and infected hundreds of thousands of people, causing substantial illness, disability or death [17–20].

This Book

This book focuses on 12 pandemics that have blighted humanity over the past 700 years. It explores three main themes: where each pandemic came from, how it spread and why it ended (if indeed it has ended). In addition, the book examines how people were affected by the pandemic, how they responded to it and the efforts made to prevent its spread of the disease. This includes the treatments, whether beneficial, ineffective or harmful, that were used. For those who wish to explore any issues in depth, each chapter provides a list of key references. These are identified in the text using superscripted numbers at the ends of paragraphs, with the full references at the end of each chapter.

Disease outbreaks begin with a few people being infected by a new disease. Mostly it ends there, as the virus or bacterium fails to spread. Only rarely does an initial outbreak become a global pandemic. It happens when several factors come together: the biology of the pathogen, the structure and organisation of society, the behaviour of populations at risk and the responses of governments. This book explores how these factors determine the global spread and the lifespan of the pandemic.

Several bodies of evidence were reviewed to identify the combination of factors responsible for each pandemic. Historical reports provide some evidence of the origin of the pandemic, the extent of disease and death and possible routes for the global spread of the disease. Reports on the social consequences of pandemics often provide evaluations of the perceived causes of the disease, the efforts made to minimise harm and the impact on people's everyday lives. Clinical studies identify the initial symptoms and long-term outcomes of infection and shed light on the ways that the disease is spread from person to person. Routinely collected data on illnesses and deaths enable epidemiological studies to explore trends in disease frequency. Finally molecular genetic studies that analyse the DNA or RNA can identify the species of the virus or bacterium, when it began infecting humans and how it has changed over time.

A final chapter summarises the findings from the 12 pandemics, contrasting the different ways in which pandemics begin, spread and end. This highlights the factors in modern civilisations that could promote the emergence of novel infectious diseases and facilitate their spread. It also identifies the strategies that could control large disease outbreaks. As pandemics have occurred with increasing frequency over the last 300 years, it seems likely that another on will emerge in the near future. This chapter emphasises the importance of being prepared to prevent and control future pandemics.

Wherever possible this book avoids technical terms. But, as this introductory chapter demonstrates, it is difficult to write about pandemics without using some of the common technical terms. These provide a concise way of presenting information, which would otherwise require lengthy explanations. Thus a short glossary is provided of key terms such as RNA, species and virus. This also prevents the wearisome repetition of explanations across the chapters.

References

1. Weiss, R. A., & Sankaran, N. (2022). Emergence of epidemic diseases: Zoonoses and other origins. *Faculty Reviews, 11*, 2.
2. Weiss, R. A. (2007). Lessons from naked apes and their infections. *Journal of Medical Primatology, 36*(4–5), 172–179.
3. Trueba, G., & Dunthorn, M. (2012). Many neglected tropical diseases may have originated in the paleolithic or before: New insights from genetics. *PLoS Neglected Tropical Diseases, 6*(3), e1393.
4. Liu, W., Li, Y., Learn, G. H., Rudicell, R. S., Robertson, J. D., Keele, B. F., et al. (2010). Origin of the human malaria parasite plasmodium falciparum in gorillas. *Nature, 467*(7314), 420–425.
5. Achtman, M. (2016). How old are bacterial pathogens? *Proceedings of the Biological Sciences, 283*(1836), 990.
6. Escalera-Zamudio, M., & Greenwood, A. D. (2016). On the classification and evolution of endogenous retrovirus: Human endogenous retroviruses may not be 'human' after all. *APMIS, 124*(1-2), 44–51.
7. Suntsova, M., Garazha, A., Ivanova, A., Kaminsky, D., Zhavoronkov, A., & Buzdin, A. (2015). Molecular functions of human endogenous retroviruses in health and disease. *Cellular and Molecular Life Sciences, 72*(19), 3653–3675.
8. Bartlett, A., Padfield, D., Lear, L., Bendall, R., & Vos, M. (2022). A comprehensive list of bacterial pathogens infecting humans. *Microbiology (Reading), 168*(12), 1269.
9. Forni, D., Cagliani, R., Clerici, M., & Sironi, M. (2022). Disease-causing human viruses: Novelty and legacy. *Trends in Microbiology, 30*(12), 1232–1242.
10. Wolfe, N. D., Dunavan, C. P., & Diamond, J. (2007). Origins of major human infectious diseases. *Nature, 447*(7142), 279–283.

11. Ehrenkranz, N. J., & Sampson, D. A. (2008). Origin of the old testament plagues: Explications and implications. *The Yale Journal of Biology and Medicine, 81*(1), 31–42.
12. Longrigg, J. (1980). The great plague of Athens. *Historia Scientiarum, 18*, 209–225.
13. Cunha, B. A. (2004). The cause of the plague of Athens: Plague, typhoid, typhus, smallpox, or measles? *Infectious Disease Clinics of North America, 18*(1), 29–43.
14. Littman, R. J., & Littman, M. L. (1973). Galen and the Antonine plague. *American Journal of Philology, 94*, 243–255.
15. Duncan-Jones, R. (2018). *The Antonine plague revisited. Arctos., 52*, 41–72.
16. Berche, P. (2022). Life and death of smallpox. *Presse Médicale, 51*(3), 104117.
17. Doshi, P. (2011). The elusive definition of pandemic influenza. *Bulletin of the World Health Organization, 89*(7), 532–538.
18. Singer, B. J., Thompson, R. N., & Bonsall, M. B. (2021). The effect of the definition of 'pandemic' on quantitative assessments of infectious disease outbreak risk. *Scientific Reports, 11*(1), 2547.
19. Morens, D. M., Folkers, G. K., & Fauci, A. S. (2009). What is a pandemic? *The Journal of Infectious Diseases, 200*(7), 1018–1021.
20. Piret, J., & Boivin, G. (2020). Pandemics throughout history. *Frontiers in Microbiology, 11*, 631736.
21. Bernstein, A. S., Ando, A. W., Loch-Temzelides, T., Vale, M. M., Li, B. V., Li, H., et al. (2022). The costs and benefits of primary prevention of zoonotic pandemics. *Science Advances, 8*(5), eabl4183.

The Black Death

There is no gentle way to introduce the Black Death; it was the deadliest of human pandemics. Sweeping across mainland Europe in 1347, it killed about one-third of the population in the following 5 years. So many people died, that it took 300 years for the population of Europe to return to pre-pandemic levels. The death rate varied substantially between countries. While Scandinavia, France, Germany, Greece and central Italy experienced high mortality, Spain, Ireland and countries in Eastern Europe were relatively spared [1–3].

As well as Europe, the disease also ravaged North Africa, the Middle East and East Asia, causing millions of deaths. The North African philosopher and historian who lived through the Black Death, Ibn Haldun, wrote of the collapse of the world order from 'a destructive plague which devastated nations and caused whole populations to vanish'. The scholar Ibn Baṭṭūṭa, an explorer and scholar, wrote of widespread disease and death as he travelled through plague-smitten lands from Iraq to Morocco. Even if these reports are exaggerated, as has been argued, the Black Death was a major scourge in North Africa and the Middle East [4–6].

Little wonder that people in the 1300s called the disease the Great Dying or the Great Pestilence. The term Black Death may derive from the Latin phrase 'atra mors' which means terrible or dreadful death. The

© The Author(s), under exclusive license to Springer Nature Singapore Pte Ltd. 2025
I. K Crombie, *Major Pandemics*, https://doi.org/10.1007/978-981-95-2081-7_2

phrase was sometimes translated black death, and this term is now widely used. The disease is also referred to as the plague. But whatever name was given to it, the process of dying was horrific [7–9].

The Process of Dying

The Black Death was caused by the bacterium *Yersinia pestis* (*Y. pestis*). It occurs in three forms: bubonic, septicaemic and pneumonic. All three forms cause symptoms of flu-like symptoms of high fever, headache and chills. These usually appear 2–3 days after infection, although it can take up to 5 or 6 days. Victims also suffer extreme weakness that makes them too exhausted to move. However, the three forms differ in other symptoms and in the length of time it takes to die [10–13].

Bubonic plague is the most common form of the infection, accounting for 70–80% of cases. Shortly after the flu-like symptoms, cases develop painful swellings of the lymph nodes, most often in the groin but also in the armpit or the neck. These swellings are commonly called buboes (from the Greek for groin) and are due to the rapid multiplication of the bacteria in lymph nodes. They can burst causing excruciating pain and spreading the bacteria throughout the body. About 60% of untreated cases die, usually within a few days of the onset of symptoms, although many survive for over a week [10–13].

The septicaemic form accounts for 10–15% of cases of plague. The bacteria enter the blood where they multiply rapidly and disrupt the coagulation system. Blood is shed from the nose, the bowels and kidneys, and it oozes into the skin, causing some blackening. Widespread blood clots lead to multiple organ failure and respiratory distress syndrome. Patients are 'struck down as if by an active poison'. About 90% of cases die within about 5 days of symptoms beginning [10, 11, 14].

Pneumonic plague, the least common form of the disease, infects the lungs. Two to 3 days after infection, the patient develops the flu-like symptoms, mild chest pain and a cough. Initially the patient produces frothy sputum, although it becomes bloody within 24 hours. Untreated, almost 100% of these with pneumonic plague die within one or 2 days of the onset of symptoms [11, 12, 15].

Reactions to the Black Death

The Black Death was catastrophic, not just for scale of death but also the impact it had on society. Petrarch, a fourteenth-century Italian philosopher and poet who lived through the Black Death, commented: 'Will you believe such things, oh posterity, when we ourselves who see them can scarcely believe them and would consider them dreams'. The writer and humanist Giovanni Boccaccio was an eyewitness to the devastation visited upon Florence in 1348. His book *The Decameron* contains searing descriptions of people behaving like animals, parents refusing to look after their children, brother abandoning brother. The sick were left to die in the streets and their bodies filled every corner. Amid the smell of decaying corpses, huge pits were dug in which bodies were stowed 'like bales of hay in the hold of a ship'. [16, 17].

Explanations for the Black Death

Christians, Muslims and Jews in Medieval times believed that plague was a punishment from God for sins committed. For Christians the sins included pride, lust, impiety and licentiousness. Many thought that the high death rate heralded the apocalypse, the end of the world and a time of the Last Judgement in which all the people who had ever lived would be assessed as virtuous or damned. Terrible disasters were thought to be a sign of the forthcoming judgement, and none more dreadful than the Black Death [18, 19].

Another theory was that cosmic forces helped the spread of Plague. In particular, the conjunction of Saturn, Jupiter and Mars was thought to poison the air which then 'contaminated the body's vital spirit and caused its organs to rot'. A related idea was that stagnant puddles and filth on city streets led to noxious disease-causing gases in the air. People became ill by inhaling the air and could transmit to others by breathing on them. As poisoned air could not be replaced, this theory gave little comfort to those living through the plague pandemic [17, 20].

In response many people resorted to prayer, fasting and religious processions through city streets to placate their wrathful god. An extreme religious group, the Flagellants, whipped themselves as they marched. This was an act of atonement for human wickedness. All the processions were initially authorised by the Pope, although they were subsequently banned when it became clear that mass gatherings were effective at spreading plague [18, 21].

Given the apparent inevitability of death, many chose to leave plague ridden towns and cities following the guidance 'Flee early, flee far, return late'. Priests and religious leaders were among those fleeing to less troubled lands. Others decided that if they were going to die, they might as well have fun and indulged in excessive eating, drinking and sexual gratification [22, 23].

The most odious response was the persecution of groups such as lepers, beggars and social minority groups, with the Jews being particularly badly treated. They were accused of spreading the disease by poisoning food and sources of water (wells and streams) in an attempt to destroy the Christian world. Some were tortured into confessing their guilt. But many more were rounded up and executed in city squares or synagogues. Those who could fled. However, although common, persecution was not universal. Many regions in France and Spain did not subscribe to the conspiracy theory, but instead tried to protect the Jews. Perhaps surprisingly, communities that suffered most from the Black Death, and those in which Jews played an important economic role were less likely to engage in persecution [24, 25].

The Black Death also contributed to major social, political and economic changes. The indiscriminate killing of apparently innocent people led many to question whether the disease was a punishment from God. This and the apparent inability of the church to control the pandemic led many to question their religion, sowing the seeds of the Reformation. In many but not all countries, labour shortages led to a rise in wages. This hastened the end of Feudalism, a system in which the peasants worked as servants or slaves, while the landlords enjoyed the wealth that was created. The ravages of the Black Death also challenged conventional views on the structure and order of society. It acted as a catalyst for the Renaissance, stimulating new approaches in philosophy, science, art and literature [17, 26, 27].

Origin and Transmission

The bacterium *Y. pestis* is thought to have evolved from a well-mannered bacterium, *Y. pseudotuberculosis*, which lived in soil and water. If eaten it causes a mild gastritis. Somewhere around 6000 years ago *Y. pestis* emerged as a new species. Several ancient skeletons, which date from 2500 to 5000 years ago, have been discovered across Europe and Asia. Analysis of bacterial DNA from these skeletons shows that *Y. pestis* infection of humans was widespread. Bacterial DNA from a 5000-year-old skeleton suggests that the plague was less infectious and caused less severe disease than more recent strains [28–30].

The strain of *Y. pestis* that caused the Black Death was a relative newcomer, only emerging in the thirteenth or early fourteenth centuries CE. This was the time of a bacteriological Big Bang, in which an ancestor strain of *Y. pestis* diverged into four new strains. One of these strains (strain 1) was responsible for the Black Death. Genetic evidence suggests that the Black Death originated in an area near the Tian Shan mountain range on the eastern border of Kyrgyzstan, a country in the centre of the Eurasian continent [31, 32].

Method of Transmission

Y. pestis is spread by the bite of the flea Xenopsylla *cheopis*. This flea lives on rodents, including rats, squirrels, marmots and prairie dogs. When a rodent dies from the infection, the fleas jump to a new host, possibly a nearby human, to obtain a continuing supply of nutritious blood. When that new host died, the flea would try to jump to another person, possibly a grieving relative [11, 33, 34].

The early strains of *Y. pestis* were poorly adapted to life in fleas. An important step in the evolution of this pathogen was the loss or inactivation of some genes and the acquisition of some new genes for increased virulence. This process probably started at least 4000 years ago, and gradually allowed the bacterium to thrive in fleas. A key development was the ability to create a slimy matrix comprising components of the blood meal and specific molecules such as proteins and polysaccharides. They clump together creating a barrier (biofilm) which blocks the flea's digestive tract, making the insect regurgitate its blood meal. Unable to digest its food, the flea repeatedly bites its host (rat or human) in a vain attempt to obtain a satisfying meal. For the bacterium this is a very effective method of ensuring it is transmitted effectively, while the poor flea dies of starvation [30, 35, 36].

The Black Death may also have been spread by the human flea *Pulex irritans* and the human louse *Pediculus humanus humanus*. These insects could acquire the disease by feeding on an infected human. Then, during close contact between humans, they could swop to new hosts spreading the disease in the process. The louse could also spread *Y. pestis* in its faeces, if these were excreted near the site of the insect bite. Scratching that itchy spot could break the skin, allowing the bacterium to enter the body and cause disease [33, 37].

One key to the success of *Y. pestis* was its ability to impair the human immune system. As humans have multiple mechanisms of inactivating invading pathogens, so the bacterium has many ways of neutralising these attacks. For example, the immune system recognises an invading bacterium and places a marker on it so that a specialised cell, a phagocyte, can destroy it. To avoid this fate, *Y. pestis* injects special proteins into the phagocyte, disrupting the normal biochemical functions so that the bacterium is not destroyed. Another technique the host uses is to sequester metal ions, such as iron and zinc, that the bacterium needs to survive. But *Y. pestis* has developed special systems that seek out the metals it requires. It seems that whatever mechanisms the host has developed to protect itself, the bacterium finds ways to evade them [29, 30, 38].

How It Spread to Europe

In 1338–1339 the first recognised outbreak of the Black Death occurred in the north of Kyrgyzstan. From the steppes of Tian Shan, it spread westwards along the Silk Road and the fur trade routes to the Middle East, Europe and North Africa. Traders and travellers passing through infected areas could have transported furs containing infected fleas or rats in sacks of grain. The initial overland travel was slow, but on reaching sea-ports the disease was quickly transported to the major European trading centres. The infection would then spread inland, usually along navigable rivers [5, 32, 39].

By 1346 the Black Death had made its way to Caffa (now called Feodosia), one of the major trading ports on the Black Sea. At that time Caffa was controlled by European merchants, although the city was under siege by the Khanate of the Golden Horde, a branch of the Mongol Empire. This army had placed an embargo on trade, preventing the ships from leaving the harbour [8, 31, 40].

The siege was abandoned when the plague arrived in the region, devastating the Mongol troops. One report suggests that the departing army used large catapults to hurl the dead bodies of plague victims into the city, hoping that the stench of corrupted air would kill those inside the walls. If true, this is probably the earliest known act of biological warfare. But the source of this story is unreliable. It is based on a report by Gabriel de' Mussi, an Italian notary who almost certainly did not witness this event. Although some commentators claim that the act of bioterrorism was a key event, others contend that it played little, if any, role in the spread of the plague [41–43].

What is true is that the lifting of the trade embargo in 1347 allowed ships to carry grain, silks, spices and the Black Death, to ports around the Mediterranean. The first ships voyaged to Messina in Sicily before travelling on to ports such as Pisa, Genoa and Marseilles. Other ships sailed directly to Egypt. Wherever the plague landed, illness and death followed. The Great Killing was underway [41, 44].

Ongoing Outbreaks of Plague

Outbreaks of the Black Death devastated Europe from 1347 to 1353, after which infection rates fell substantially for a time. But for the next 400 years waves of plague spread across Europe and the Middle East about every 10–12 years, some causing substantial mortality. In total, just over 6500 outbreaks of plague occurred in Europe from 1347 to the early 19th century [5, 33, 45].

These outbreaks were most likely caused by repeated reintroduction of the disease from outside Europe. It is thought that reservoirs of plague among rodents living in Central Asia were the source of the reinfections. The unanswered question is what stimulated these sporadic reimportations. One suggestion is that climate changes in Central Asia caused the populations of rodents and their fleas to expand rapidly. This substantially increased the risk of the infection being transmitted by rodents to humans journeying along trade routes [46].

Given the frequency of outbreaks of plague, there was obvious interest in knowing when next one was beginning. In the sixteenth century, London developed a system of counting the number of deaths from plague for each parish (local community). These were compiled centrally so that the progress of outbreaks could be monitored. Initially only senior figures in local government had access to the information which was used to establish where quarantine should be imposed. The City Watch (essentially a police force) sealed up houses containing plague victims, preventing residents from leaving. To warn others to stay away, the front door was then marked with a white cross. However, people clamoured for information on plague outbreaks because it would let them know when it was time to flee. As a result, printed summaries of recent plague deaths were posted in markets and on churches [47–49].

The plague outbreaks of 1623–1632 and 1647–1657 were particularly severe, affecting much of Western Europe. The 30 Years War (1618–1648) may have been a major factor in the spread of disease across the continent. One notable outbreak was the Great Plague which struck London and much of the rest of England in 1665. It began quietly with two deaths in Drury Lane just before Christmas 1664, followed by 6 weeks during which no deaths from plague were reported. Then further deaths occurred, with the numbers rapidly increasing from February to reach a peak in October. After this, deaths gradually declined so that by January 1666 the outbreak was over. It is estimated that some 70,000 people had died, about 15% of the population of London [26, 50, 51].

When the village of Eyam in Derbyshire suffered an outbreak in 1665, it responded with an extraordinary act of altruism. A batch of clothes ordered from London by local tailor contained fleas infected with plague. As people became ill, the local vicar, William Mompesson, persuaded the villagers to seal themselves off to prevent spread to the surrounding areas. When the outbreak had run its course, 267 of the villagers had died, some 80% of the population. Even the vicar's wife Catherine had succumbed to the infection. Her tomb is preserved in the local cemetery. Sadly, the villagers' decision to seal themselves off may have led to the very high death rate [52, 53].

The outbreaks in the mid-1600s could suggest that the plague was still rampaging across Europe, but in fact it had been in decline from about 1640. The eighteenth century witnessed only two major outbreaks: in Marseille in 1720 and in Moscow in 1770–1771. Only some minor outbreaks occurred in the 19th century [54, 55].

The Other Two Plague Pandemics

The Black Death was not the first plague pandemic. That unwanted honour is given to the Plague of Justinian, named after the man who was the Roman Emperor when the plague struck in 541 CE. Historical sources suggest that this plague originated in India, travelled to East Africa and then to Egypt, around the Mediterranean Basin and into Europe. However genetic studies suggest it could also have originated in Central Asia [40, 56, 57].

The first the Romans knew about this pandemic was an outbreak of plague at the Egyptian port of Pelusium in the Nile delta in 541 CE. The disease spread through Syria and Turkey reaching Greece and Italy by the spring of 542, and eventually as far as Ireland in 544. Every part of the Roman Empire was blighted by this pandemic. Constantinople, the capital city of this empire, is thought to have suffered most. At the height of this outbreak some 10,000 people died each day, and up to half of the population had died by the time the plague abated [58, 59].

The initial wave subsided in 544 CE, but was followed by subsequent waves every 8–12 years until about 750 CE. None was as severe as the initial outbreak. Estimates of the total deaths over the 200 or so years of this plague vary widely from a few hundred thousand to 100 million. Many of the early estimates are thought to have greatly exaggerated the numbers who died. This plague may have contributed to the fall of the Roman Empire [40, 59–61].

The Third Plague Pandemic

Not satisfied with two pandemics, *Y. pestis* has caused a third one. It began in the Yunnan province south-west China in 1772 and travelled slowly to reach Hong Kong in 1894. On hearing the news about this outbreak, several scientists rushed to the plague-stricken regions to study the disease. Among them was Alexander Yersin, who identified the bacterium which caused plague. In his honour it was named *Yersinia pestis* (Yersin had initially named it *Pasteurella pestis* after the pioneering microbiologist Louis Pasteur). The mechanism of spread of the disease, from the bite of an infected rat flea, was established by Paul-Louis Simond, a French physician who worked on outbreaks in India and Pakistan in 1897 and 1898. His published results were initially met with scepticism, until other researchers confirmed the findings [62, 63].

From Hong Kong the disease spread to Singapore and Bombay in 1896 and was then carried around the world by steamships. The port cities of Sidney, Honolulu, Vera Cruz, Capetown, Alexandria and Glasgow were among those infected. Because of extensive railway networks, the plague also ventured far inland. However, in contrast to the Black Death, the global death toll was low, although many deaths occurred in the densely populated regions of India, China and Indonesia. Thus, while cities such as Glasgow, San Francisco, and Honolulu recorded fewer than one hundred cases between 1894 and 1901, Hong Kong and had over 2000. India probably suffered most harm with an estimated 13 million deaths over the period 1898–1949 [4, 33, 64].

When Did the Black Death End?

The Black Death only lasted from 1347 to 1353, but it was followed by many waves of plague. These outbreaks only stopped in the early decades of the nineteenth century, so it is fair to say that this plague lasted for almost 500 years. However, the dates at which it ended varied greatly across the countries across Europe. Plagues had mostly disappeared from Italy in 1650 and from England in the 1670s. France experienced its last outbreak in 1720, but plagues continued in Southeastern Europe until 1840 [34, 55, 65].

Several explanations have been put forward for the gradual disappearance of these outbreaks. One possibility is that the bacterium mutated to become less virulent. Genetic studies have provided some evidence to support this, although it is fragmentary and far from being conclusive. There is evidence against this view: the outbreaks in the sixteenth and seventeenth centuries were as virulent as those in the fourteenth and fifteenth centuries. This suggests there was no systematic decline in virulence [55].

Another possibility is that rats which were susceptible to plague were gradually killed by infection with *Y. pestis*. This would select for rats which were resistant to the plague. These surviving rats would be unable to pass the bacterium to uninfected fleas, interrupting the cycle of transmission. This proposal has a weakness. It does not easily explain why many towns and cities had repeated outbreaks over hundreds of years. If the susceptible rats were killed after the first or second outbreaks, what was sustaining the subsequent rounds of the infection [33, 34, 65].

A more likely explanation for the decline in outbreaks is the increased use of widely enforced quarantine, particularly at the major ports. This could have prevented the spread of the infection. The system of quarantine as a means to control the Black Death was first developed in the city of Ragusa (modern-day Dubrovnik) in 1377. Initially ships arriving at the port had to anchor offshore for a 30-day isolation period. This was extended to 40 days because the shorter period did not prevent the spread of disease. The measure was also applied to land travellers. The Italian term for this interval, quaranta giorno (literally 40 days), is the origin of the word quarantine [55, 65–67].

The city of Ragusa introduced another measure to reduce the spread of disease. It established a place to care for plague victims, and those suspected of having the disease. They were housed in buildings outside the city walls. This reduced the risk of the disease being spread to near neighbours. Other cities gradually adopted these practices: Marseille in 1383,

Venice in 1423, Pisa (1464) and Genoa (1467). Venice took this further in 1423, by creating the world's first hospital for plague victims, which was located on a nearby island. The widespread use of quarantine and the isolation of cases might explain why Italy was one of the first countries to be free of plague [22, 65, 68].

The gradual improvement of housing stock by the use of brick and stone to construct buildings could also have contributed to the decline of plague. These buildings would be more rat-resistant than the earlier houses which were wooden and had thatched roofs. This was best seen following the Great Fire of London in 1665, where the wood/thatch houses were replaced by those built of brick. Afterwards there were no more outbreaks of plague in London. It could be that the black rat, which played a major role in spreading plague, much preferred to live in the fabric of the wooden buildings. This rat could have been replaced by the sewer-dwelling brown rat. It preferred to living away from humans and would be less likely to pass on its fleas. But the building of brick houses cannot easily explain why the plague disappeared at different times in different places. At best the structure of houses only plays a part in the ending of this disease [65, 67].

Finally, there is an explanation that focuses on Kyrgyztan, the source of the repeated waves of plague that devastated the Middle East, Europe and North Africa. It is suggested that these outbreaks resulted from particular climatic conditions that greatly increased the number of fleas infected with plague. This makes it more likely that traders travelling on the Silk Road would encounter these fleas and carry the disease westward. However, if the appropriate climatic conditions occurred less frequently, then there would be fewer outbreaks of plague in the Middle East, Europe and North Africa. There is some evidence to support this view [46, 54, 69].

The true explanation of how this plague ended may never be known. It seems likely that the use of quarantine, the building of brick houses and favourable climatic conditions contributed to the eventual disappearance of plague outbreaks in the nineteenth century. But that is not the end of the story; the plague is still with us.

Reservoirs and Re-emergence

The worldwide spread of plague during the third pandemic has established reservoirs of infection in Southeast Asia, Africa, North and South America. The favoured, or rather unfortunate, regions are those with high altitude, a warm and dry climate and a ready supply of susceptible rodents. In these locations rodents regularly undergo large fluctuations in population size, depending on climate, food availability, presence of predators and land use changes. Their tendency to live close to human products such as crops and waste material, helps promote rodent numbers and increase the risk of disease transmission [70–72].

Madagascar has recently suffered from several instances of plague re-emergence from reservoirs. Steamboats from India transported *Y. pestis* to the island in 1898, and it became established in central regions above 800 metres. Madagascar suffered two large outbreaks in the early 1900s, after which infections subsided to low levels. However large outbreaks resumed in the mid-1990s, and in 2004, 2013 and 2017. Tanzania and the Democratic Republic of Congo experienced similar disease patterns to Madagascar, with small outbreaks being followed by a few large ones, then a gradual diminution in the number of cases. Currently, Madagascar and the Democratic Republic of Congo report most cases of plague [73–75].

Localised outbreaks of plague will continue, but a major pandemic is very unlikely. There is a slim chance that it could happen if a virulent new strain of pneumonic plague emerged. A large outbreak of the highly infectious form of plague struck Manchuria, north-east China, in 1910. The outbreak was explosive because it was being spread by respiratory aerosols. More than 50,000 people died. It was brought under control as a result of international efforts to implement preventive measures such as border controls, quarantine and mask wearing. By itself such an outbreak could not cause a major pandemic. It would need to be combined with several other destructive events such as wars, cataclysmic earthquakes and major tsunamis. Then amidst the chaos, and the determination of people to flee quickly and far, a new plague pandemic might spread globally. The odds of these happening at the same time are vanishingly small [76, 77].

References

1. Zietz, B. P., & Dunkelberg, H. (2004). The history of the plague and the research on the causative agent Yersinia pestis. *International Journal of Hygiene and Environmental Health, 207*(2), 165–178.
2. Izdebski, A., Guzowski, P., Poniat, R., Masci, L., Palli, J., Vignola, C., et al. (2022). Palaeoecological data indicates land-use changes across Europe linked to spatial heterogeneity in mortality during the black death pandemic. *Nature Ecology & Evolution, 6*, 297–306.
3. Pamuk, S. (2007). The black death and the origins of the 'great divergence' across Europe, 1300–1600. *European Review of Economic History, 11*, 289–317.
4. Echenberg, M. (2002). Pestis redux: The initial years of the third bubonic plague pandemic, 1894-1901. *Journal of World History, 13*, 429–449.
5. Dols, M. W. (1979). The second plague pandemic and its recurrences in the Middle East: 1347-1894. *Journal of the Economic and Social History of the Orient, 22*(2), 162–189.
6. Tresso, C. (2021). A two-year journey under the arrows of the black death: The medieval plague pandemic in Ibn Baṭṭūṭa's travels. *Journal of Arabic and Islamic Studies, 21*, 137–189.
7. Why, V. N., & Death, I. B. (2021). Black? European gothic imaginaries of 'oriental' plague. In C. Lynteris (Ed.), *Plague image and imagination from medieval to modern times. Medicine and biomedical sciences in modern history* (pp. 11–35). Palgrave Macmillan.
8. McEvedy, C. (1988). The bubonic plague. *Scientific American, 258*(2), 118–123.
9. Frith, J. (2012). The history of plague - part 1: The three great pandemics. *J Military Veterans Health., 20*, 11–16.
10. Cantlie, J. (1900). The signs and symptoms of bubonic, pneumonic, and Septicaemic plague. *British Medical Journal, 2*(2078), 1229–1232.
11. Rosario Acevedo, R., Biryukov, S. S., Bozue, J. A., & Cote, C. K. (2021). Plague prevention and therapy: Perspectives on current and future strategies. *Biomedicine, 9*(10), 1421.
12. Kugeler, K. J., Staples, J. E., Hinckley, A. F., Gage, K. L., & Mead, P. S. (2015). Epidemiology of human plague in the United States, 1900-2012. *Emerging Infectious Diseases, 21*(1), 16–22.
13. Sebbane, F., & Lemaître, N. (2021). Antibiotic therapy of plague: A review. *Biomolecules, 11*(5), 724.

14. Riedel, S. (2005). Plague: From natural disease to bioterrorism. *Baylor University Medical Center Proceedings, 18*(2), 116–124.
15. Pechous, R. D., Sivaraman, V., Stasulli, N. M., & Goldman, W. E. (2016). Pneumonic plague: The darker side of Yersinia pestis. *Trends in Microbiology, 24*(3), 190–197.
16. Wojciehowski, D. (2005). Francis petrarch: First modem friend. *Texas Studies in Literature and Language, 47*, 269–298.
17. Getz, F. M. (1991). Black death and the silver lining: Meaning, continuity, and revolutionary change in histories of medieval plague. *Journal of the History of Biology, 24*(2), 265–289.
18. Stearns, J. (2009). New directions in the study of religious responses to the black death. *History Compass., 7*, 1–13.
19. The, L. R. (1981). Black death and Western European eschatological mentalities. *The American Historical Review, 86*, 533–552.
20. Henderson, J. (2020). The invisible enemy: Fighting the plague in early modern Italy. *Centaurus, 62*, 263–274.
21. Tuchman, B. (1978). *"This is the end of the world": the black Death. A distant mirror: The calamitous fourteenth century* (pp. 98–133). Penguin Random House.
22. Porter, R. (1999). *The greatest benefit to mankind.* Harper Collins.
23. Khan, I. A. (2004). Plague: The dreadful visitation occupying the human mind for centuries. *Transactions of the Royal Society of Tropical Medicine and Hygiene, 98*(5), 270–277.
24. Cohn, S. (2012). Pandemics: Waves of disease, waves of hate from the plague of Athens to a.I.D.S. *Historical Research, 85*, 535–555.
25. Jedwab, R., Johnson, N., & Koyama, M. (2019). Negative shocks and mass persecutions: evidence from the black death. *Journal of Economic Growth, 24*, 346–395.
26. Alfani, G., & Murphy, T. (2017). Plague and lethal epidemics in the pre-industrial world. *The Journal of Economic History, 77*, 314–343.
27. Moore, J. (2002). The crisis of feudalism: An environmental history. *Organization and Environment, 15*, 301–322.
28. Susat, J., Lübke, H., Immel, A., Brinker, U., Macāne, A., Meadows, J., et al. (2021). A 5,000-year-old hunter-gatherer already plagued by Yersinia pestis. *Cell Reports, 35*(13), 109278.
29. Demeure, C. E., Dussurget, O., Mas Fiol, G., Le Guern, A. S., Savin, C., & Pizarro-Cerdá, J. (2019). Yersinia pestis and plague: An updated view on

evolution, virulence determinants, immune subversion, vaccination, and diagnostics. *Genes and Immunity, 20*(5), 357–370.
30. Andrades Valtueña, A., Neumann, G. U., Spyrou, M. A., Musralina, L., Aron, F., Beisenov, A., et al. (2022). Stone age Yersinia pestis genomes shed light on the early evolution, diversity, and ecology of plague. *Proceedings of the National Academy of Sciences of the United States of America, 119*(17), e2116722119.
31. Green, M. (2020). How a microbe becomes a pandemic: A new story of the black death. *Lancet, 1*, e311–e3e2.
32. Spyrou, M. A., Musralina, L., Gnecchi Ruscone, G. A., Kocher, A., Borbone, P. G., Khartanovich, V. I., et al. (2022). The source of the black Death in fourteenth-century Central Eurasia. *Nature, 606*(7915), 718–724.
33. Barbieri, R. (2021). Origin, transmission, and evolution of plague over 400 y in Europe. *Proceedings of the National Academy of Sciences of the United States of America, 118*(39), e2114241118.
34. Appleby, A. (1980). The disappearance of plague: A continuing puzzle. *The Economic History Review, 33*, 161–173.
35. Hinnebusch, B. J., Jarrett, C. O., & Bland, D. M. (2017). "Fleaing" the plague: Adaptations of Yersinia pestis to its insect vector that lead to transmission. *Annual Review of Microbiology, 71*, 215–232.
36. Spyrou, M. A., Tukhbatova, R. I., Wang, C. C., Valtueña, A. A., Lankapalli, A. K., Kondrashin, V. V., et al. (2018). Analysis of 3800-year-old Yersinia pestis genomes suggests bronze age origin for bubonic plague. *Nature Communications, 9*(1), 2234.
37. Walløe, L. (2008). Medieval and modern bubonic plague: Some clinical continuities. *Medical History. Supplement, 27*, 59–73.
38. Price, S. L., Vadyvaloo, V., DeMarco, J. K., Brady, A., Gray, P. A., Kehl-Fie, T. E., et al. (2021). Yersiniabactin contributes to overcoming zinc restriction during Yersinia pestis infection of mammalian and insect hosts. *Proceedings of the National Academy of Sciences of the United States of America, 118*(44), e2104073118.
39. Yue, R. P. H., Lee, H. F., & Wu, C. Y. H. (2017). Trade routes and plague transmission in pre-industrial Europe. *Scientific Reports, 7*(1), 12973.
40. Barbieri, R., Signoli, M., Chevé, D., Costedoat, C., Tzortzis, S., Aboudharam, G., et al. (2020). Yersinia pestis: The natural history of plague. *Clinical Microbiology Reviews, 34*(1), e00044.
41. Barker, H. (2021). Laying the corpses to rest: Grain, embargoes, and Yersinia pestis in the Black Sea, 1346–48. *Speculum, 96*, 97–126.

42. Wheelis, M. (2002). Biological warfare at the 1346 siege of Caffa. *Emerging Infectious Diseases, 8*(9), 971–975.
43. Ditrich, H. (2017). The transmission of the black Death to western Europe: A critical review of the existing evidence. *Mediterranean Historical Review, 32*, 25–39.
44. Watts, S. (1997). The human response to plague in Western Europe and the Middle East, 1347-1844. In *Epidemics and history: Disease, power and imperialism* (pp. 1–39). Yale University Press.
45. Stenseth, N. C., Tao, Y., Zhang, C., Bramanti, B., Büntgen, U., Cong, X., et al. (2022). No evidence for persistent natural plague reservoirs in historical and modern Europe. *Proceedings of the National Academy of Sciences of the United States of America, 119*(51), e2209816119.
46. Schmid, B. V., Büntgen, U., Easterday, W. R., Ginzler, C., Walløe, L., Bramanti, B., et al. (2015). Climate-driven introduction of the black Death and successive plague reintroductions into Europe. *Proceedings of the National Academy of Sciences of the United States of America, 112*(10), 3020–3025.
47. Heitman, K. (2020). Authority, autonomy and the first London bills of. *Mortality, 62*, 275–284.
48. Robertson, J. (1996). Reckoning with London: Interpreting the bills of mortality before John Graunt. *Urban History., 23*, 325–350.
49. Ogle, W. (1892). An inquiry into the trustworthiness of the old bills of mortality. *Journal. Royal Statistical Society, 55*, 437–460.
50. Glatter, K. A., & Finkelman, P. (2021). History of the plague: An ancient pandemic for the age of COVID-19. *The American Journal of Medicine, 134*(2), 176–181.
51. Sloan, A. W. (1973). Medical and social aspects of the great plague of London in 1665. *South African Medical Journal, 47*(7), 270–276.
52. Massad, E., Coutinho, F. A., Burattini, M. N., & Lopez, L. F. (2004). The Eyam plague revisited: did the village isolation change transmission from fleas to pulmonary? *Medical Hypotheses, 63*(5), 911–915.
53. Whittles, L. K., & Didelot, X. (2016). Epidemiological analysis of the Eyam plague outbreak of 1665-1666. *Proceedings of the Biological Sciences, 283*(1830), 20160618.
54. Eckert, E. A. (2000). The retreat of plague from Central Europe, 1640-1720: A geomedical approach. *Bulletin of the History of Medicine, 74*(1), 1–28.
55. Stenseth, N., Dear, K., & Brammanti, B. (2022). The end of plague in Europe. *J Europ Soc Hist Sci., 64*, 61–72.

56. Keller, M., Spyrou, M. A., Scheib, C. L., Neumann, G. U., Kröpelin, A., Haas-Gebhard, B., et al. (2019). Ancient Yersinia pestis genomes from across Western Europe reveal early diversification during the first pandemic (541-750). *Proceedings of the National Academy of Sciences of the United States of America, 116*(25), 12363–12372.
57. Pisarenko, S. V., Evchenko, A. Y., Kovalev, D. A., Evchenko, Y., Bobrysheva, O. V., Shapakov, N. A., et al. (2021). Yersinia pestis strains isolated in natural plague foci of Caucasus and Transcaucasia in the context of the global evolution of species. *Genomics, 113*(4), 1952–1961.
58. The, A. P. (1979). Justinian. *Plague. Byzantion., 49*, 5–20.
59. Sarris, P. (2021). New approaches to the 'plague of Justinian'. *Past & Present., 254*, 315–346.
60. Perry, R. D., & Fetherston, J. D. (1997). Yersinia pestis–etiologic agent of plague. *Clinical Microbiology Reviews, 10*(1), 35–66.
61. Mordechai, L., Eisenberg, M., Newfield, T. P., Izdebski, A., Kay, J. E., & Poinar, H. (2019). The justinianic plague: An inconsequential pandemic? *Proceedings of the National Academy of Sciences of the United States of America, 116*(51), 25546–25554.
62. Simond, M., Godley, M. L., & Mouriquand, P. D. (1998). Paul-Louis Simond and his discovery of plague transmission by rat fleas: A centenary. *Journal of the Royal Society of Medicine, 91*(2), 101–104.
63. Hinnebusch, B. J. (2012). Biofilm-dependent and biofilm-independent mechanisms of transmission of Yersinia pestis by fleas. In A. de Almeida & N. Leal (Eds.), *Advances in Yersinia research. 954* (pp. 237–243). Springer.
64. Bramanti, B., Dean, K. R., Walløe, L., & Chr, S. N. (1901). The third plague pandemic in Europe. *Proceedings of the Biological Sciences, 2019*(286), 20182429.
65. Slack, P. (1981). The disappearance of plague: An alternative view. *The Economic History Review, 34*, 469–476.
66. Tognotti, E. (2013). Lessons from the history of quarantine, from plague to influenza a. *Emerging Infectious Diseases, 19*(2), 254–259.
67. Slack, O. (2022). End of a pandemic? contemporary explanations for the end of plague in 18th-century England. *Centaurus, 64*(1), 87–98.
68. Gensini, G. F., Yacoub, M. H., & Conti, A. A. (2004). The concept of quarantine in history: From plague to SARS. *The Journal of Infection, 49*(4), 257–261.
69. Yue, R. P. H., & Lee, H. F. (2020). Drought-induced spatio-temporal synchrony of plague outbreak in Europe. *Sci Total Environ., 698*, 134138.

70. Mahmoudi, A., Kryštufek, B., Sludsky, A., Schmid, B. V., Lei, X., et al. (2021). Plague reservoir species throughout the world. *Integrative Zoology, 16*(6), 820–833.
71. Zeppelini, C. G., de Almeida, A. M., & Cordeiro-Estrela, P. (2016). Zoonoses as ecological entities: A case review of plague. *PLoS Neglected Tropical Diseases, 10*(10), e0004949.
72. Ecke, F., Han, B. A., Hörnfeldt, B., Khalil, H., Magnusson, M., Singh, N. J., et al. (2022). Population fluctuations and synanthropy explain transmission risk in rodent-borne zoonoses. *Nature Communications, 13*(1), 7532.
73. Chanteau, S., Ratsifasoamanana, L., Rasoamanana, B., Rahalison, L., Randriambelosoa, J., Roux, J., et al. (1998). Plague, a reemerging disease in Madagascar. *Emerging Infectious Diseases, 4*(1), 101–104.
74. Alderson, J., Quastel, M., Wilson, E., & Bellamy, D. (2020). Factors influencing the re-emergence of plague in Madagascar. *Emerging Topics in Life Sciences, 4*(4), 411–421.
75. Bertherat, E. (2019). Plague around the world in 2019. *Weekly Epidemiological Record, 25*, 289–292.
76. Michaleas, S. N., Laios, K., Karamanou, M., Sipsas, N. V., & Androutsos, G. (2022). The Manchurian pandemic of pneumonic plague (1910-1911). *Le Infezioni in Medicina, 30*(3), 464–468.
77. Levison, M. E. (2000). Lessons learned from history on mode of transmission for control of pneumonic plague. *Current Infectious Disease Reports, 2*(4), 269–271.

Syphilis

Introduction

The syphilis pandemic began towards the end of 1494 when the French king Charles VIII was planning to invade Italy. At that time a few of his troops had become infected with the syphilis bacterium. The army invaded and quickly occupied Rome and Naples. After this easy victory, the soldiers engaged in extended carousing and debauchery involving prostitution and rape. Although they were unaware of it, frequent sexual intercourse results in the rapid spread of syphilis. A few months later many of the troops became ill with an eruption of spots across their bodies. These were 'boils that stood out like acorns, from whence issued such filthy stinking matter' [1–3].

Handicapped by illness, the army of Charles VIII was defeated at the battle of Fornovo in July 1495. The demoralised troops, who were mainly mercenaries, disbanded and returned to their various homelands carrying syphilis across Europe. The infection reached France, Germany and Switzerland by the end of 1495, and then Holland and Greece in 1496. The following year it arrived in England and Scotland, and by 1499 Hungary and Russia experienced outbreaks of syphilis. European sailors then transported it around the known world, where it caused outbreaks

© The Author(s), under exclusive license to Springer Nature Singapore Pte Ltd. 2025

I. K Crombie, *Major Pandemics*, https://doi.org/10.1007/978-981-95-2081-7_3

in India and China in the early 1500s. Seldom have two battles led to a major pandemic [1, 2].

Since that first outbreak, hundreds of millions of people have been infected with syphilis. Among the many unknown victims are several notable historical figures, including royalty (Ivan the Terrible and Henry VIII), writers (John Keats and Oscar Wilde), musicians (Beethoven and Schubert) and artists (Goya and van Gogh) [3, 4].

Early Names

Syphilis has been given a variety of names. At first it was simply called a cruel pestilence (peste cruelle) or an unknown pestilence (ignota pestis) because it was a new disease. Subsequently the term 'the Great Pox' was used, describing boils the size of acorns on the victim's skin. (The term 'pox' is an old English word for a pimple.) This label was also used to distinguish the disease from smallpox, a pandemic characterised by small spots. Syphilis was also named Lues Venerea (venereal plague) after Venus the Roman goddess of love [5].

The term 'syphilis' was coined in 1530 by the Italian poet, doctor and scholar Girolamo Fracastoro a few years after the pandemic began. In his poem 'Syphilis sive morbus gallicus' (Syphilis or the French disease) he relates how a shepherd called Syphilus annoyed the god Apollo by worshiping a local king instead of the god. As punishment, Apollo inflicted a hideous disease, syphilis, on the local population. The poem, which provides a clear description of the disease, was widely read in countries such as Italy, Germany and England. They took the opportunity to blame the French for spreading the disease, adopting the name morbus gallicus. In response the French called it the Neapolitan disease because the first major outbreak was in Naples. Other countries followed the tradition of blaming the neighbours, with the Russians labelling it the Polish disease, and those in Poland calling it the German disease. As the disease spread eastwards, the Turkish called it the Christian disease, and in north India the Hindus and Moslems blamed each other, until both groups united in blaming the Europeans. This pattern of name shaming has earned syphilis the title of 'the most disowned infection in history' [2, 6, 7].

The Discovery of the Bacterium

The cause of syphilis was identified during the golden age of bacteriology. Pioneering research by Louis Pasteur and Robert Koch had shown that diseases could be caused by bacteria, tiny single-celled organisms that could be seen in a microscope. In the late 1800s this led to a fevered hunt for the microbial causes of diseases. Although many false claims were made, the search was successful in the case of syphilis. The first step was to confirm that syphilis was infectious. This was achieved by taking material from a patient with syphilis and injecting it into several great apes in 1903. These unfortunate animals were successfully infected. Then 2 years later, two doctors, Schaudinn and Hoffman, examined material taken from a papule on a woman with secondary syphilis. Under the microscope they saw a strange new long, thin, spiral bacterium now named *Treponema pallidum* (subspecies pallidum). It is often called a spirochete, because of its spiral form and its method of moving by corkscrewing around. Initially there was doubt about the finding, but this was quickly overcome when other scientists confirmed the result [8, 9].

The Disease and Its Complications

The first sign of infection is a small, raised spot, often called a chancre or ulcer, at the site where the bacterium entered the body. It can appear on the genitals, the anus or the mouth, depending on which part of the body has been in contact with the chancre of an infected person. These spots are readily visible on the penis but are less likely to be seen within the folds of skin around the vagina or on the anus, so many people may be unaware that they have been infected [10–12].

The initial spot usually appears some three to 4 weeks after intercourse; it is firm and painless, although sometimes a fluid oozes from it. Wherever it emerges, the spot disappears within a few weeks, possibly giving a false sense of relief to the individual. In reality, the bacterium has spread to tissues throughout the body within a few hours of infection [12–15]..

The second stage appears from a few weeks up to 3 months later. Most of those infected (50–70%) develop red or brown blotchy rashes, usually on the palms of the hands or the soles of the feet, although they can occur elsewhere on the body. Patients often experience flu-like symptoms, such as fever, headache, joint pains and tiredness. Usually these symptoms pass within a few weeks. Some patients also experience neurological symptoms such as stiff neck, blurred vision, hearing loss and mental confusion [12, 14].

About one-third of those infected progress to the final stage of the disease sometime between 2 and 20 years after the initial infection. Healthy tissues are damaged by the destructive effects of fleshy growths or nodules that are composed of syphilis bacteria and white blood cells. These mainly affect the skin and the bones but can also cause damage in other organs; for example, about 10% of those with third stage disease develop serious cardiovascular problems. Most unpleasant are the neurological complications that develop 5–10 years after the initial infection. These include personality changes, loss of memory, hallucinations and loss of sight. Patients with such symptoms were once given the diagnosis general paralysis of the insane and were cared for by psychiatrists. It is now known that all the symptoms of final stage of syphilis infections are a consequence of the immune response that the body mounts in an unsuccessful attempt to rid itself of the bacterium [14, 16].

Treatments Old and New

The early treatments for syphilis were mostly ineffective and almost always harmful. Initially, conventional therapies such as bloodletting were used. A flowering plant from the Americas (guaiac) quickly gained a reputation as a cure for syphilis. Also known as 'sacred wood' or 'wood of life', it was thought to be effective against skin diseases. However, it fell out of favour as evidence emerged that it failed to cure the infection. Another approach was to apply hot irons to the visible sores causing considerable pain but having no effect on the progress of the infection. Possibly the most popular treatment was the use of the toxic metal mercury in a variety of concoctions. The cause of the disease and the duration of treatment are captured in the phrase: 'Two minutes with venus, two years with mercury'. Mercury induced the production of copious amounts of phlegm which in theory carried away the poison causing the disease. There were two indications that the treatment was thought to be working: when the patient could spit out at least three pints of phlegm a day, and when their teeth started to fall out [17–19].

An antibiotic to treat syphilis was discovered in the early twentieth century. Paul Ehrlich, a German biochemist, had spent many years searching for a 'magic bullet' that could destroy pathogenic microorganisms. He focused on arsenic, a toxic metal that had often been used to poison kings and emperors. By combing it with other chemicals he tried to produce a compound that could kill microorganisms without doing too much harm to humans. After testing 605 compounds Ehrlich finally succeeded with the 606th. It was named Salvarsan, from the Latin 'salvare' to save, and was hailed as a wonder drug for the treatment of syphilis. Although this drug was much better than the early remedies, it had toxic side effects. It also had to be taken weekly for a year or more [20–22].

In contrast to Salvarsan, penicillin was discovered by chance in 1929. But as Louis Pasteur observed, 'chance favours the prepared mind'. The man who stumbled on penicillin was Alexander Fleming. He was studying staphylococcal bacteria and was clearing out a collection dishes on which the bacteria had been grown. Then he stopped suddenly, remarking, 'that's funny'. On one of the dishes, no bacteria were growing near a colony of the mould (*Penicillium notatum*). Intrigued by finding he correctly reasoned that a chemical produced by the mould was killing the bacteria. He named it penicillin, but despite many attempts he was unable to isolate the active ingredient. Other scientists who attempted to extract the chemical also failed, and *Penicillium notatum* was ignored [23].

Then in 1937 a team of researchers in Oxford led by Howard Florey and Ernst Chain focused their efforts on extracting penicillin. By 1940 they succeeded and showed that it could treat bacterial infections in mice. The problem was that their crude extracts were not suitable for large-scale use in humans; attempts at purification only yielded enough material to treat one or two people. At this time the Second World War was underway, making it essential to provide sufficient quantities of pure penicillin to treat wounded soldiers. Florey moved to the United States as it had the resources to develop methods to mass-produce penicillin. By 1943 there were sufficient supplies of the drug to treat all the allied troops. Penicillin was a godsend, and in 1945 Fleming, Florey and Chain were awarded the Nobel Prize for their work. But there is a footnote. A research team in Peoria, Illinois, screened 1000 samples of the mould and found that only three produced large amounts of penicillin. What are the chances that 1 day Fleming would stumble on one of those three strains on one culture dish among a pile that were being cleared out? [23].

Theories of Origin

The emergence of a disease that began to ravage populations in 1495 led to many interesting theories about its cause. A common view was that it was inflicted by God who was angry at the sinful behaviour of human beings. Possibly it appeared fitting that promiscuity was punished by a disease spread by sexual intercourse. Woodcuts and paintings from 1496 illustrated the painful sores with which immoral behaviours were punished. Astrological explanations also flourished. The conjunction (alignment) of Mars, Jupiter and Saturn in 1484 was held responsible for the appearance of this new disease. A variation on this theme held that Venus, the planet associated with the goddess of love, exerted a power which could transmute an old disease into a virulent new one [2, 5, 17].

There is consensus among researchers that the syphilis pandemic began in Italy in 1495, but there is disagreement about its origins. Some say that the first pandemic of syphilis was all the fault of that man Columbus. He was looking for a westward route to Asia, but instead discovered the Caribbean islands. While there, some of his crew are thought to have contracted syphilis from the local inhabitants. They brought the disease back to Europe on their return in 1493. This is supported by reports from Spanish doctors that some of Columbus' sailors did suffer from a strange unknown disease. As syphilis spread across Europe, there were many reports of a new and very unpleasant disease that was spread by sexual intercourse. Syphilis had arrived in Europe [2, 24, 25].

An alternative view, the pre-Columbian hypothesis, is that syphilis had existed in Europe for many years before Columbus went sailing. Studies of ancient bacterial DNA obtained from human remains suggest that syphilis could have been present in Europe before Columbus sailed to the New World. However, there are too few samples of ancient bacterial DNA to support or refute any of the hypotheses. Another theory was that syphilis evolved from other closely related diseases such as yaws and bejel (caused by bacteria very closely related to syphilis). This appears plausible as the DNA of the bacteria that cause these diseases is 99.8% identical to that of syphilis. It is also possible that syphilis was not recognised because it was misdiagnosed as other diseases such as leprosy. Because there is insufficient evidence to confirm any of the theories, the origin of syphilis remains unresolved [26, 27].

Spread of the Disease

Syphilis is mainly spread by sexual intercourse. It is often called a stealth pathogen, because of the ease with which it evades the host's immune system. The outer membrane of the spirochete has evolved so that it contains very few targets for the defensive antibodies to recognise. That property, together with its ability to spread rapidly throughout the body, makes syphilis a highly successful parasite [28].

Syphilis is infectious during the first and second stages of the disease (from the initial appearance of the chancre to the disappearance of the red and brown blotches). This means that an infected person can spread the disease for up to 3 or 4 months. The risk of contracting syphilis depends on who you have sex with, how often you do so and how many sexual contacts your partner has recently had. It is difficult to put an exact figure on the risk. One study concluded that the disease will be transmitted to about 50–60% of sexual contacts with an infected person. A more recent study found that about one-third of all sexual contacts will successfully transmit syphilis. In a sense an exact figure is unnecessary; having sex with someone in the early stages of syphilis is really not a good idea [29, 30].

Long-Term Trends in Infection Rates

The frequency of syphilis infections has varied greatly since the pandemic began at the end of the fifteenth century. All countries have seen marked fluctuations in the numbers of new cases. Sometimes groups of countries will have infection rates that follow similar trajectories, but many will experience changes in disease frequency that are due to factors unique to them. Three large countries—the United States, China and the former Soviet Union—have discordant trends that result from the effects of different political, social and economic factors. Exploring these trends can help identify the reasons for the present high rates of infection [31].

United States

Wars are particularly effective at increasing sexually transmitted disease rates among soldiers and subsequently in civilian populations. The United States has experienced several spikes in the rates of syphilis among American soldiers in wars between 1840 and 1918: the Mexican War (1846–1848), the Civil War (1861–1866), the Spanish-American War (1898) and the First World War (1914–1918). However, once the wars were over, the rates subsided as quickly as they had risen [31].

Possibly the most dramatic fall in the rates of syphilis infection occurred at the end of the Second World War. From a peak of almost 80 new cases per 100,000 population in 1945, it had tumbled to 5 cases per 100,000 in 1952. Much of the reduction could be due to the fall in cases that always follows shortly after the end of hostilities, but penicillin also played a part. This newly available effective treatment was delivered through the creation of countrywide treatment centres, supplemented by active searching for new cases. Syphilis was under control [32].

But things changed in America in the 1960s. It was the time of the civil rights movement, hippies, the summer of love and the counterculture movement. This was accompanied by a marked liberalisation of attitudes to sexual behaviour in the 1960s and early 1970s. Perhaps not surprisingly, the increase in syphilis infections began in the late 1950s and plateaued at 12 new cases per 100,000 in the mid-1960s. From 1963 to 1978 the rates fluctuated, although the underlying trend was to higher rates in men and lower rates in women. The increase in male rates was partly due to cases among men who have sex with men (MSM) [32–34].

With increasing awareness of the dangers of the HIV/AIDS epidemic in the late 1980s, the rates of syphilis among men and women fell for the next decade. When a new highly effective treatment for AIDS was developed in the late 1990s, the fear of catching HIV abated. This probably resulted in a higher frequency of sexual activity because the rates of new cases among men began to rise, reaching 25 per 100,000 by 2022. The increase in men was largely driven by high-risk behaviours among men who have sex with men, such as illicit drug use, multiple partners and unprotected anal intercourse. However, there was also an increase in heterosexual cases [35–37].

A major feature of syphilis in the United States is the variation in infection rates between the racial groups. Many factors contribute to these differences, particularly access to healthcare, poverty and cultural attitudes to sex. Although syphilis cases have fluctuated over time in America, people of African origin have always experienced substantially higher infection rates than all other racial groups. Currently their rates are almost five times higher than those of whites, although in previous years the disparity has been much greater. Most of the other racial groups (Hispanic, American Indians/Native Alaskans, Native Hawaiians/Pacific Islanders and Multirace) have intermediate infection rates. Only Asians have lower rates than whites [32, 38–40].

China

China is notable for the way in which strong political action controlled one epidemic of syphilis and health promotion campaigns failed to deal with a second. The disease was first brought to China by Portuguese traders in the early 1500s. Syphilis became widespread, but data on the frequency of infection was sparse until the 1930s and 1940s, when an estimated 5% of city dwellers and 2–3% of those in rural areas had syphilis. Prostitution was widespread at that time, with up to 50% of female sex workers carrying the infection [41].

The situation changed dramatically when Mao Zedong came to power in 1949. In a national plan to improve the health of the poor, sexually transmitted diseases were branded as an evil Western influence. To redress this, brothels were closed, prostitution was criminalised and a nationwide programme of screening and treatment was implemented. By 1964 China was declared syphilis-free. That state continued until 1979 when, following the death of Mao Zedong, a programme of economic reform opened its borders to Western visitors. There was also an increased tolerance of extramarital sex and of commercial sex workers. The numbers of cases began to rise again [41, 42].

In response the Chinese government identified the 'Six Evils': commercial sex work, pornography, trafficking women, dealing and using drugs, gambling and profiting from superstition. To tackle these evils it launched a massive educational campaign in 1991. This had little effect. Instead, the frequency of infection rose 25-fold between 1991 and 1998. And it got worse; from 1999 to 2009 the number of cases increased from 72,000 to 150,000. This prompted the creation of a national syphilis control plan in 2010. It involved intensive screening of people attending healthcare and those in high-risk groups (female sex workers and MSM). It was effective. By 2016 case numbers subsided to just over 100,000, and data up to 2020 confirm the continuing impact of this programme [43–46].

Russia

After the breakup of the Soviet Union in 1991, the newly formed Russian Federation experienced a rapid rise in syphilis cases. Between 1990 and 1997 the rate of infections in Russia rose 50-fold, from 5.4 to 266.9 per 100,000. Many of newly independent countries of the former Soviet Union experienced similar large increases rates. These increases were a consequence of the social and economic disruption that followed the disintegration of the Soviet Union. GDP (gross domestic product) fell, inflation was high and the real value of wages fell. The result was a sharp drop in standards of living and large increases in unemployment, particularly among women. Poverty was widespread, and Russia became one of the most economically unequal countries in the world. In addition, sex was glamorised, pornography was widely available and prostitution thrived. Casual sexual contacts were common and syphilis spread rapidly at a time when a reduction in spending on healthcare meant there were fewer facilities for treatment and prevention [47–49].

Injecting drug use was another major factor in the rapid increase in syphilis. When Afghanistan substantially increased its heroin production in the late 1980s, it used Russia as a major transport route to Europe. Given the widespread poverty, drug dealing became a useful source of income and drug use provided an escape from the harsh living conditions. The increase in supply led to a fall in price and a rapid increase in heroin addiction. Sharing needles and syringes was a common practice among drug users in Russia. It is also an efficient method of spreading syphilis because of the residual amounts of blood in used equipment. Women who inject drugs often exchange sex for drugs, engaging in unprotected vaginal intercourse and sharing drug using equipment [49–51].

The impact of the major economic shocks appeared to be relatively short lived: from the peak of 266.9 per 100,000 in 1997, the rates in Russia fell to 79 per 100,000 in 2004 and to 29 per 100,000 in 2013. The rates in the other former Soviet Union countries experienced similar reductions. Syphilis has now become concentrated in minority groups: the homeless, those in detention facilities, sex workers and injecting drug users [52, 53].

The Current Global Situation

In 2022 there were an estimated eight million new cases of syphilis. However, the frequency of disease varies substantially across the regions of the world. The lowest rate is in Central Asia (43 per 100,000 population), whereas that in Central sub-Saharan Africa is more than 20 times higher at 1048 per 100,000. Broadly speaking the rates are low in Europe, Australasia, the United States and Canada, North Africa and Central Asia (range between 43 and 84 per 100,000). Moderate rates, in the range 100–250 per 100,000, are found in Latin America, the Caribbean, and

South and South-East Asia. Rates above 400 per 100,000 only occur in sub-Saharan Africa and Oceania [54, 55].

The high rates of syphilis in sub-Saharan Africa are partly driven by HIV infection. People who are HIV-positive are at a much higher risk of contracting syphilis. This is because the HIV virus greatly weakens the immune system, allowing the syphilis bacterium to thrive. What makes things worse is that syphilis infection greatly increases the risk of contracting HIV. It is thought that syphilitic ulcers damage the skin, allowing the HIV virus to enter the body [56, 57].

Although their rates are low, syphilis in high-income countries is currently on the increase. Across Europe the overall number of infections rose steadily between 2007 and 2017, and was largely driven by increases among men who have sex with men. In five countries (Iceland, Ireland, the UK, Germany and Malta) the rates of infection more than doubled over this 11-year period. This trend of increased rates in Europe has continued to 2021. In the United States the number of cases increased by 74% between 2017 and 2021. Canada experienced a five-fold increase in the frequency of syphilis between 2011 and 2020. In Australia case numbers rose from 1719 in 2013 to 6063 in 2022 [58–63].

Congenital Syphilis

A distressing feature of this disease is congenital syphilis. The bacterium *Treponema pallidum* can cross the placenta of pregnant women to infect the unborn foetus. About two-thirds of pregnant women with active syphilis will transmit the disease to their foetuses. Just over half of the babies that have the infection experienced adverse birth outcomes. One-third of them die from it. The good news is that the serological test for syphilis in pregnancy will detect almost all cases of infection, and treatment with the antibiotic penicillin is a very effective cure [64].

The World Health Organization has identified congenital syphilis as a high priority for action. In theory, screening pregnant women for syphilis and treating those infected with antibiotics should prevent congenital syphilis. However, in many countries attendance at antenatal clinics is poor and screening for syphilis is often not carried out. In addition, some of those found to be infected are not treated. Two technical difficulties contribute to these problems: insufficient procurement of screening kits and the limited availability of the appropriate antibiotic. Resolving these issues will be difficult. Even in a high-income country like the United States, lack of timely antenatal care and lack of appropriate treatment are major barriers to the prevention of congenital syphilis [65–67].

For a few years interventions to reduce congenital syphilis appeared to be working: the number of cases per 100,000 live births fell from 540 cases in 2012 to 473 cases in 2016. Since then rates have risen to 523 cases of congenital syphilis per 100,000 live births in 2022. WHO has set targets of <200 per 100,000 live births in 2025 and <50 for 2030. These are very unlikely to be met. The reality is that only half of pregnant women with syphilis receive treatment. Also worrying is that middle- and high-income countries, which can afford high-quality antenatal care, have recently experienced large increases in the number of syphilis infections in pregnancy. Congenital syphilis is a serious problem that is getting worse [54, 64].

Control Measures

As there is no vaccine to prevent infection, the main method of syphilis control is with diagnostic tests and the highly effective treatment penicillin. It requires attendance at a clinic to conduct the screening test and to administer the drug by injection. As the needle has to be pushed into a muscle, it can be painful. This combination of factors can discourage attendance. Provision of discreet access to screening services could improve syphilis detection rates. An alternative would be to supply self-testing kits. These kits are less expensive than testing in clinics and have high levels of acceptability among high-risk groups. But there is no alternative to attending clinics for the injection [68–70].

Tracing the contacts of individuals who test positive to syphilis can also help reduce the spread of syphilis. This requires clinics to ask attendees to disclose the names and contact details of their sexual partners. There is a marked reluctance to provide this information, so many of these individuals are not treated. More worrying is that the methods of syphilis control, screening and contact tracing, will have limited impact on low- and middle-income countries. They often lack the necessary surveillance systems and laboratory testing facilities for syphilis control, and services such as discreet clinics and self-testing kits may not be available [71–73].

The oldest method of preventing syphilis transmission, apart from abstinence, is the use of condoms. They were initially made from the intestines of sheep, calves or goats, but this was replaced by rubber in 1855 and by latex in the 1930s. The limitations are that people may be reluctant to buy or to use them, and sometimes they slip off during intercourse. They are most effective when used consistently, something that may be difficult in the heat of the moment [29, 74].

Another method of preventing syphilis is pre-exposure prophylaxis (PrEP) and post-exposure prophylaxis (PEP). This uses the antibiotic doxycycline, which is taken as a tablet. Individuals who are about to, or have recently, engaged in high-risk activities take this antibiotic to prevent syphilis infection. PEP is highly effective and has been licensed for use in Canada and the United States. But PreEP is more problematic, as it may encourage anal sex which greatly increases the risk of infection. There is also the concern that a high-frequency use of drugs such as doxycycline could result in the development of antibiotic resistance [75–77].

Behaviour change interventions to reduce the frequency of risky sexual behaviour have had mixed results. Intensive efforts can help pregnant woman avoid congenital syphilis in their babies, but men who have sex with men are much more resistant to change. There is some evidence that nationwide mass communication campaigns can reduce the number of reported cases of syphilis [78–80].

Reducing infection rates in high-risk groups, sex workers, injecting drug users and people in prison is particularly challenging. The reasons are obvious: sex workers have multiple partners, drug users often share dirty needles and prisoners can also have multiple sexual partners. Behaviour change interventions are being developed for these groups, but it is far from certain that they will have a major impact on infection rates [80, 81].

The development of an effective vaccine against syphilis could provide the key to controlling infection rates. Work on such a vaccine began shortly after the identification of the bacterium *T. pallidum* in the early years of the twentieth century. More than 100 years later the sought-after vaccine remains elusive. The main problem is that the outer membrane of the virus provides very few targets for the immune system to attack. So far 'a practical and effective vaccine formulation continues to elude scientists' [82, 83].

When Will the Pandemic End?

After 500 years of widespread infection, syphilis remains a serious problem. Effective treatments have been available for more than 70 years, but the number of new cases of syphilis and congenital syphilis is currently increasing. The spread of syphilis is a result of the biological drive to procreate, greatly aided by the recent liberalisation of attitudes to sexual intercourse. It has become more common to have multiple sexual partners. Mobile apps and internet chat rooms make it much easier to identify new partners and expand sexual networks.

In 2016 the World Health Organization launched a campaign to reduce the global number of the cases of syphilis by 90% by 2030. It was scheduled to begin in 2018 when there were six million new cases. By 2020 the number had risen to 7.1 million from where it increased to 8 million in 2022. An interim target for 2025 was to reduce the number of cases to 5.7 million by 2025, with the final target of 0.71 million in 2030. It seems very unlikely that these ambitious aims will be achieved [54, 65].

There are many control measures that can help reduce infection rates. But what seems to be lacking is commitment from governments, backed up by adequate resources, to implement intervention campaigns on national scales. Possibly there is insufficient political will to intervene in the sexual activities of the general population. The decisive action taken by the Chinese authorities in 1949 was certainly effective, but few countries would be willing to replicate those measures today.

The problem is that tackling high-risk sexual behaviours raises a conflict between individual rights to sexual freedom and the state's responsibility for the health and welfare of all its citizens. Just how much effort can be made to encourage individuals to alter their sexual behaviour without it becoming coercive? The issue becomes more problematic with groups such as female sex workers, men who have sex with men and people in prisons. Across the world they have high rates of rates of syphilis. But what types of intervention are fair to these individuals and also reduce the risk of infection in the wider community? [84].

WHO has set out five strategic directions to control syphilis. These cover delivering high-quality healthcare, optimising systems and partnerships, using data to drive decisions, empowering communities and fostering innovations. Within each of these directions, many key topics and important professional and societal groups are identified. What the report lacks is a clear specification of who will take the initiative, what actions they will take, how will they manage conflicting views on the best course of action and where the funding to support these activities will come from [66].

It is easy to be critical of WHO when it is confronted with what is essentially a messy problem: one that is inherently complex, involves multiple stakeholders who have different goals and requires significant judgement (i.e. there is considerable uncertainty about the impact of any actions taken). Improved healthcare, better diagnostic tests and an effective vaccine would certainly help, but it is not clear when these will become available. At present, there is no indication of how or when the syphilis pandemic will end.

References

1. Tognotti, E. (2009). The rise and fall of syphilis in renaissance Europe. *The Journal of Medical Humanities, 30*(2), 99–113.
2. Tampa, M., Sarbu, I., & Georgescu, S. (2014). Brief history of syphilis. *Journal of Medicine and Life, 7*, 4–10.
3. Bowater, L. (2016). The great pox. *Microbiology Today, 43*, 178–181.
4. Wright, A. D. (1971). Venereal disease and the great. *The British Journal of Venereal Diseases, 47*(4), 295–306.
5. Abel, E. (2018). Syphilis: the history of an eponym. *Names A Journal of Onomastics, 66*, 96–102.

6. Spitzer, L. (1955). The etymology of the term syphilis. *Bulletin of the History of Medicine, 29*(3), 269–273.
7. Ross, J. J. (2005). Shakespeare's chancre: Did the bard have syphilis? *Clinical Infectious Diseases, 40*(3), 399–404.
8. Rivers, T. M. (1937). Viruses and Koch's postulates. *Journal of Bacteriology, 33*(1), 1–12.
9. de Souza, E. (2005). A hundred years ago, the discovery of Treponema pallidum*. *Anais Brasileiros de Dermatologia, 80*, 547–548.
10. Anonymous. (2004). Transmission of primary and secondary syphilis by oral sex--Chicago, Illinois, 1998–2002. *MMWR. Morbidity and Mortality Weekly Report, 53*(41), 966–968.
11. Ghanem, K. G., Ram, S., & Rice, P. A. (2020). The modern epidemic of syphilis. *The New England Journal of Medicine, 382*(9), 845–854.
12. Nyatsanza, F., & Tipple, C. (2016). Syphilis: Presentations in general medicine. *Clinical Medicine (London, England), 16*(2), 184–188.
13. Singh, A. E., & Romanowski, B. (1999). Syphilis: Review with emphasis on clinical, epidemiologic, and some biologic features. *Clinical Microbiology Reviews, 12*(2), 187–209.
14. Lafond, R. E., & Lukehart, S. A. (2006). Biological basis for syphilis. *Clinical Microbiology Reviews, 19*(1), 29–49.
15. Goh, B. T. (2005). Syphilis in adults. *Sexually Transmitted Infections, 81*(6), 448–452.
16. Waddington, K., Thomas, R., & Willis, M. (2011). General paralysis of the insane. *Practical Neurology, 11*(6), 366–369.
17. Kikuchihara, Y., & Hirai, H. (2022). Syphilis in renaissance medicine. In M. Sgarbi (Ed.), *Encyclopaedia of renaissance philosophy* (pp. 3181–3183). Springer International Publishing.
18. Abraham, J. J. (1948). Some account of the history of the treatment of syphilis. *The British Journal of Venereal Diseases, 24*(4), 153–161.
19. O'Shea, J. G. (1990). 'Two minutes with venus, two years with mercury'--mercury as an antisyphilitic chemotherapeutic agent. *Journal of the Royal Society of Medicine, 83*(6), 392–395.
20. Frith, J. (2013). Arsenic—the "poison of kings" and the "saviour of syphilis". *Journal of Military and Veterans' Health, 21*, 11–17.
21. Parascandola, J. (2001). John Mahoney and the introduction of penicillin to treat syphilis. *Pharmacy in History, 43*(1), 3–13.

22. Bosch, F., & Rosich, L. (2008). The contributions of Paul Ehrlich to pharmacology: A tribute on the occasion of the centenary of his Nobel prize. *Pharmacology, 82*(3), 171–179.
23. Ligon, B. L. (2004). Penicillin: Its discovery and early development. *Seminars in Pediatric Infectious Diseases, 15*(1), 52–57.
24. Morton, R. S. (1968). Another look at the morbus gallicus. Postscript to the meeting of the medical society for the study of venereal diseases, Geneva, may 26-28, 1967. *The British Journal of Venereal Diseases, 44*(2), 174–177.
25. Baker, B. J., Crane-Kramer, G., Dee, M. W., Gregoricka, L. A., Henneberg, M., Lee, C., et al. (2020). Advancing the understanding of treponemal disease in the past and present. *American Journal of Physical Anthropology, 171*(Suppl 70), 5–41.
26. Beale, M. A., & Lukehart, S. A. (2020). Archaeogenetics: What can ancient genomes tell us about the origin of syphilis? *Current Biology, 30*(19), R1092–R1095.
27. Majander, K., Pfrengle, S., Kocher, A., Neukamm, J., du Plessis, L., Pla-Díaz, M., et al. (2020). Ancient bacterial genomes reveal a high diversity of treponema pallidum strains in early modern Europe. *Current Biology, 30*(19), 3788–3803.e10.
28. Radolf, J. D., Deka, R. K., Anand, A., Šmajs, D., Norgard, M. V., & Yang, X. F. (2016). Treponema pallidum, the syphilis spirochete: Making a living as a stealth pathogen. *Nature Reviews. Microbiology, 14*(12), 744–759.
29. Stoltey, J. E., & Cohen, S. E. (2015). Syphilis transmission: A review of the current evidence. *Sexual Health, 12*(2), 103–109.
30. Denman, J., Hodson, J., & Manavi, K. (2022). Infection risk in sexual contacts of syphilis: A systematic review and meta-analysis. *The Journal of Infection, 84*(6), 760–769.
31. Idsoe, O., & Guthe, T. (1967). The rise and fall of the treponematoses. I. ecological aspects and international trends. in venereal syphilis. *The British Journal of Venereal Diseases, 43*(4), 227–243.
32. Nakashima, A. K., Rolfs, R. T., Flock, M. L., Kilmarx, P., & Greenspan, J. R. (1996). Epidemiology of syphilis in the United States, 1941--1993. *Sexually Transmitted Diseases, 23*(1), 16–23.
33. Ashbolt, A. (2018). We can be together: Hippie culture as radical community. *Counterculture Studies, 1*, 48–63.
34. Thornton, A., & Young-DeMarco, L. (2001). Four decades of trends in attitudes toward familyissues in the United States: The 1960s through the 1990s. *Journal of Marriage and the Family, 63*, 1009–1037.

35. Peterman, T. A., Su, J., Bernstein, K. T., & Weinstock, H. (2015). Syphilis in the United States: on the rise? *Expert Review of Anti-Infective Therapy, 13*(2), 161–168.
36. Centre for Disease Control and Prevention. (2024). *Sexually transmitted disease surveillance 2022.* U.S. Department of Human Health Services. https://www.cdc.gov/std/statistics/2022/overview.htm
37. Schmidt, R., Carson, P. J., & Jansen, R. J. (2019). Resurgence of syphilis in the United States: An assessment of contributing factors. *Infectious Diseases, 12*, 1178633719883282.
38. Patton, M. E., Su, J. R., Nelson, R., & Weinstock, H. (2014). Primary and secondary syphilis—United States, 2005-2013. *MMWR. Morbidity and Mortality Weekly Report, 63*(18), 402–406.
39. Centers for Disease Control and Prevention. (2019). *Sexually transmitted disease surveillance 2018.* CDC.
40. Centers for Disease Control and Prevention. (2021). *Sexually transmitted disease surveillance 2019.* CDC.
41. Hesketh, T., Ye, X., & Zhu, W. (2008). Syphilis in China: The great comeback. *Emerging Health Threats Journal, 1*, e6.
42. Lin, C. C., Gao, X., Chen, X. S., Chen, Q., & Cohen, M. S. (2006). China's syphilis epidemic: A systematic review of seroprevalence studies. *Sexually Transmitted Diseases, 33*(12), 726–736.
43. Abrams, H. K. (2001). The resurgence of sexually transmitted disease in China. *Journal of Public Health Policy, 22*(4), 429–440.
44. Chen, X. S., Gong, X. D., Liang, G. J., & Zhang, G. C. (2000). Epidemiologic trends of sexually transmitted diseases in China. *Sexually Transmitted Diseases, 27*(3), 138–142.
45. Tao, Y., Chen, M. Y., Tucker, J. D., Ong, J. J., Tang, W., Wong, N. S., et al. (2020). A nationwide spatiotemporal analysis of syphilis over 21 years and implications for prevention and control in China. *Clinical Infectious Diseases, 70*(1), 136–139.
46. Shi, L., Chen, L., Liu, X., Hu, H., Chen, Y., Chen, Y., et al. (2023). Evaluating the effect of the plan of national syphilis control in controlling the syphilis epidemic in Jiangsu, China 2010-2020. *Frontiers in Public Health, 11*, 1281229.
47. Netesov, S. V., & Conrad, J. L. (2001). Emerging infectious diseases in Russia, 1990-1999. *Emerging Infectious Diseases, 7*(1), 1–5.

48. Riedner, G., Dehne, K. L., & Gromyko, A. (2000). Recent declines in reported syphilis rates in eastern Europe and Central Asia: are the epidemics over? *Sexually Transmitted Infections, 76*(5), 363–365.
49. Radcliffe, K. (2005). Developing evidence-based guidelines for the management of sexually transmitted diseases in former Soviet Union countries. *International Journal of STD & AIDS, 16*(9), 589–593.
50. Rhodes, T., Platt, L., Maximova, S., Koshkina, E., Latishevskaya, N., Hickman, M., et al. (2006). Prevalence of HIV, hepatitis C and syphilis among injecting drug users in Russia: A multi-city study. *Addiction, 101*(2), 252–266.
51. Benotsch, E., Somlai, A., Pinkerton, S., et al. (2004). Drug use and sexual risk behaviours among female Russian IDUs who exchange sex for money or drugs. *International Journal of STD & AIDS, 15*, 343–347.
52. Bailey, H., Turkova, A., & Thorne, C. (2017). Syphilis, hepatitis C and HIV in Eastern Europe. *Current Opinion in Infectious Diseases, 30*(1), 93–100.
53. Shakarishvili, A., Dubovskaya, L. K., Zohrabyan, L. S., St Lawrence, J. S., Aral, S. O., Dugasheva, L. G., et al. (2005). Sex work, drug use, HIV infection, and spread of sexually transmitted infections in Moscow. *Russian Federation. Lancet., 366*(9479), 57–60.
54. World Health Organization. (2024). *Implementing the global health sector strategies on HIV, viral hepatitis and sexually transmitted infections, 2022–2030: report on progress and gaps 2024*. World Health Organization.
55. Du, M., Yan, W., Jing, W., Qin, C., Liu, Q., Liu, M., et al. (2022). Increasing incidence rates of sexually transmitted infections from 2010 to 2019: An analysis of temporal trends by geographical regions and age groups from the 2019 global burden of disease study. *BMC Infectious Diseases, 22*(1), 574.
56. Wu, M. Y., Gong, H. Z., Hu, K. R., Zheng, H. Y., Wan, X., & Li, J. (2021). Effect of syphilis infection on HIV acquisition: A systematic review and meta-analysis. *Sexually Transmitted Infections, 97*(7), 525–533.
57. Marchese, V., Tiecco, G., Storti, S., Degli Antoni, M., Calza, S., Gulletta, M., et al. (2022). Syphilis infections, reinfections and serological response in a large Italian sexually transmitted disease Centre: A monocentric retrospective study. *Journal of Clinical Medicine, 11*(24), 7499.
58. European Centre for Disease Prevention and Control. (2019). *Syphilis and congenital syphilis in Europe—A review of epidemiological trends (2007–2018) and options for response*. ECDC.
59. Mitjà, O., Padovese, V., Folch, C., Rossoni, I., Marks, M., Rodríguez, I. A. M. A., et al. (2023). Epidemiology and determinants of reemerging

bacterial sexually transmitted infections (STIs) and emerging STIs in Europe. *The Lancet Regional Health, 34*, 100742.

60. Centre for Disease Control and Prevention. (2023). *Sexually transmitted disease surveillance 2023*. Centre for Disease Control and Prevention. https://www.cdc.gov/std/statistics/2021/default.htm
61. Aho, J., Lybeck, C., Tetteh, A., Issa, C., Kouyoumdjian, F., Wong, J., et al. (2022). Rising syphilis rates in Canada, 2011-2020. *Canada Communicable Disease Report, 48*(23), 52–60.
62. UK Health Security Agency. (2023). *Sexually transmitted infections (STIs): annual data tables*. UK Government. https://www.gov.uk/government/statistics/sexually-transmitted-infections-stis-annual-data-tables
63. Aung, E., & Chow, E. (2024). Testing and capturing difficult-to-access populations for syphilis control in Australia. *Microbiology Australia, 45*(3), 142–146.
64. Korenromp, E. L., Rowley, J., Alonso, M., Mello, M. B., Wijesooriya, N. S., Mahiané, S. G., et al. (2019). Global burden of maternal and congenital syphilis and associated adverse birth outcomes-estimates for 2016 and progress since 2012. *PLoS One, 14*(2), e0211720.
65. World Health Organization. (2018). *Report on global sexually transmitted infection surveillance 2018*. World Health Organization.
66. World Health Organization. (2022). *Global health sector strategies on, respectively, HIV, viral hepatitis and sexually transmitted infections for the period 2022–2030*. WHO.
67. Taylor, M., Gliddon, H., Nurse-Findlay, S., Laverty, M., Broutet, N., Pyne-Mercier, L., et al. (2018). Revisiting strategies to eliminate mother-to-child transmission of syphilis. *The Lancet Global Health, 6*(1), e26–ee8.
68. Stamm, L. V. (2015). Syphilis: Antibiotic treatment and resistance. *Epidemiology and Infection, 143*(8), 1567–1574.
69. Singh, A. (2019). How to address the resurgence of syphilis in Canada. *CMAJ, 191*, E1367–E1368.
70. Towns, J. M., Tieosapjaroen, W., Mello, M. B., Baggaley, R. C., Johnson, C. C., Jamil, M. S., et al. (2023). The role of syphilis self-testing as an additional syphilis testing approach in key populations: A systematic review and meta-analysis. *The Lancet Public Health, 8*(9), e726–ee34.
71. Golden, M. R., Gibbs, J., Woodward, C., & Estcourt, C. S. (2022). Priorities in the implementation of partner services for HIV/STIs in high-income nations: A0 narrative review of evidence and recommendations. *Sexual Health, 19*(4), 309–318.

72. Moseley, P., Bamford, A., Eisen, S., Lyall, H., Kingston, M., Thorne, C., et al. (2024). Resurgence of congenital syphilis: New strategies against an old foe. *The Lancet Infectious Diseases, 24*(1), e24–e35.
73. Martin, K., Wenlock, R., Roper, T., Butler, C., & Vera, J. H. (2022). Facilitators and barriers to point-of-care testing for sexually transmitted infections in low- and middle-income countries: A scoping review. *BMC Infectious Diseases, 22*(1), 561.
74. Marfatia, Y. S., Pandya, I., & Mehta, K. (2015). Condoms: Past, present, and future. *Indian Journal of Sexually Transmitted Diseases and AIDS, 36*(2), 133–139.
75. Cornelisse, V. J., Riley, B., & Medland, N. A. (2024). Australian consensus statement on doxycycline post-exposure prophylaxis (doxy-PEP) for the prevention of syphilis, chlamydia and gonorrhoea among gay, bisexual and other men who have sex with men. *The Medical Journal of Australia, 220*(7), 381–386.
76. Szondy, I., Meznerics, F. A., Lőrincz, K., Kemény, L. V., Walter, A., Mohammed, A. A., et al. (2024). Doxycycline prophylaxis for the prevention of sexually transmitted infections: A systematic review and meta-analysis of randomized controlled trials. *International Journal of Infectious Diseases, 147*, 107186.
77. Hart, T. A., Noor, S. W., Berlin, G. W., Skakoon-Sparling, S., Tavangar, F., Tan, D., et al. (2023). Pre-exposure prophylaxis and bacterial sexually transmitted infections (STIs) among gay and bisexual men. *Sexually Transmitted Infections, 99*(3), 167–172.
78. Peterman, T. A., & Cha, S. (2018). Context-appropriate interventions to prevent syphilis: A narrative review. *Sexually Transmitted Diseases, 45*(9S Suppl 1), S65–S71.
79. Paiva, J. C. L., Dias-Trindade, S., Gonzalez, M. O. A., Barros, D., Cardoso, P. H., Bezerra, P. H. C., et al. (2022). Analysis of the impact of communication campaigns under the project "syphilis no": A national tool for inducing and promoting health. *International Journal of Environmental Research and Public Health, 19*(23), 15884.
80. de Wit, J. B. F., Adam, P. C. G., den Daas, C., & Jonas, K. (2023). Sexually transmitted infection prevention behaviours: Health impact, prevalence, correlates, and interventions. *Psychology & Health, 38*(6), 675–700.
81. Ong, J. J., Fu, H., Smith, M. K., & Tucker, J. D. (2018). Expanding syphilis testing: A scoping review of syphilis testing interventions among key populations. *Expert Review of Anti-Infective Therapy, 16*(5), 423–432.

82. Kojima, N., Konda, K. A., & Klausner, J. D. (2022). Notes on syphilis vaccine development. *Frontiers in Immunology, 13*, 952284.
83. Li, S., Li, W., Jin, Y., Wu, B., & Wu, Y. (2023). Advancements in the development of nucleic acid vaccines for syphilis prevention and control. *Human Vaccines & Immunotherapeutics, 19*(2), 2234790.
84. Miller, A. M., Kismödi, E., Cottingham, J., & Gruskin, S. (2015). Sexual rights as human rights: A guide to authoritative sources and principles for applying human rights to sexuality and sexual health. *Reproductive Health Matters, 23*(46), 16–30.

Yellow Fever

Introduction

Yellow fever was once a feared disease and remains an ongoing cause of illness and death. It was commonly called Yellow Jack because a yellow flag (a jack) was often raised to warn people when the fever had been detected. As the disease could spread rapidly, the flag was seen as a warning that illness and death awaited travellers to an infected area. In the seventeenth century, yellow fever was often carried by members of the crews of sailing ships. This may have inspired the legend of the Flying Dutchman, a ship that inhabited by the ghosts of sailors who had died from the infection. It was doomed to roam the seas for eternity because no port would allow entry to a vessel infested with this deadly disease. Other terms for yellow fever include black vomit and black blood, symptoms of a severe form of the disease. The disease caused fear because outbreaks often began without warning, rampaging through towns and cities for weeks or months, killing up to 10% of the population. Then it would disappear as quickly as it started, only to reappear several years later. This fear was made worse because no one knew how yellow was spread [1, 2].

© The Author(s), under exclusive license to Springer Nature Singapore Pte Ltd. 2025

I. K Crombie, *Major Pandemics*, https://doi.org/10.1007/978-981-95-2081-7_4

The Virus and the Infection

Yellow fever is caused by an RNA virus. It belongs to a group of about 70 viruses called flaviviruses. (Flavi means yellow and the group was named after its most prominent member, yellow fever.) Several other flaviviruses cause serious illness, particularly dengue virus, Japanese encephalitis virus, Omsk haemorrhagic fever, West Nile virus and tick-borne encephalitis virus. As their names imply, the prominent symptoms can be haemorrhagic disease, encephalitis, fever, paralysis and jaundice [3].

Not everyone who is infected suffers severe illness or death. Most people, about 55% of those infected, have either no symptoms at all or experience very mild ones. A further 33% develop a flu-like illness with headache, widespread muscle pain, dizziness and general unwellness. This lasts for about 3 days then the patient recovers. The remaining 12% are less fortunate. They have the same initial flu-like symptoms but then, after an apparent remission lasting a few hours, the fever returns. This time it is accompanied by nausea, jaundice (the yellow skin colour that gave the disease its name), internal bleeding, vomiting of blood and damage to the liver, kidneys and the heart. Up to half of those with severe disease die from the infection die within 10 days of the onset of the new symptoms. To date there is no effective treatment for yellow fever, but those who survive the disease have lifelong immunity to further infection [4–6].

The Early Outbreaks

The first recorded outbreak of yellow fever was in 1648 in the Yucatan Peninsula (southeast Mexico) and was most likely a continuation of the disease that had struck Barbados in 1647. From the Yucatan the infection spread throughout the Caribbean then gradually faded away. The next confirmed epidemic began in states on Brazil's Atlantic coast, first in Pernambuco in 1685 and then in Bahia the following year. After over 150 years of relative quiet, interrupted by a few handfuls of cases, the next serious outbreak in Brazil began in Bahia state in 1849. It then spread to Rio de Janeria where over 4000 people died [7, 8].

The coastal cities of the United States, such as Boston, New York, Charleston and New Orleans, suffered repeated attacks of the disease from 1693 to 1905. A particularly large outbreak devastated Philadelphia in 1793 killing 10,000 people, about 9% of the population. Possibly the worst outbreak in the Americas was in the Mississippi Valley in 1878. About 20,000 people died in the towns and cities between Memphis and New Orleans. In contrast, Europe was relatively spared, although major Mediterranean ports such as Cadiz, Malaga Barcelona and Marseille were afflicted on several occasions. Even English ports, Swansea and Southampton, had the occasional outbreak [9–11].

Outbreaks and the Louisiana Purchase

A yellow fever outbreak most likely played a major part in the 1803 Louisiana Purchase. This was a political deal by which the American government acquired a vast swathe of land in central North America. For the sum of $15 million it doubled the amount of territory it occupied. The history of the events leading up to this purchase is complex, with France, Spain and Britain constantly vying for control of territories in North America and the Caribbean islands. A key event was the battle for St Domingue, present-day Haiti. In 1802 Napoleon Bonaparte sent a fleet of 86 ships and 30,000 men to invade St Domingue with the aim establishing a lucrative colony based on exporting sugar to Europe. This was first step of a grand plan that Napoleon had devised. The next stage was to strengthen and expand the territories that the French held in North America [12, 13].

The French army initially made progress against the local troops in St Dominique, but then faced an ongoing guerrilla war. What made things substantially worse was the number of fatalities from yellow fever among French soldiers. Estimates of the proportion who died are high, ranging from 40% to 80%. The French were unfortunate to have mounted an invasion during a particularly severe yellow fever outbreak. The catastrophic losses limited Napoleon's ability to establish a grand empire in the Americas. He also had to contend with a possible alliance between America and Britain that would result in war if France tried to expand its territories in North America. Napoleon withdrew from the region, having decided to switch his focus to the domination of Europe. As a result, America acquired a vast new territory that included New Orleans, the key sea port for the lucrative Mississippi river trade. Seldom has one country acquired so much land without a shot being fired [12, 13].

How Yellow Fever Is Transmitted

For over 250 years there was an ongoing and vigorous debate between the supporters of the two theories of disease causation: miasma and contagion. Proponents of the miasma explanation thought that the disease resulted from corrupted gases emanating from rotting organic matter. But this theory cannot explain why the noxious vapours were present in the summer months every year, whereas outbreaks of yellow fever occurred at irregular intervals several years apart. The contagionists believed that the disease was passed from directly person to person. However, this couldn't explain why healthy people could contract the disease without having had any contact with an infected individual. More telling, healthcare staff who looked after the severely ill patients seldom contracted the disease. Without an understanding of how it was spread, people were helplessness in the face major outbreaks of disease [1, 2, 7, 14].

It wasn't until the early years of the twentieth century that the method of transmission of yellow fever was finally unravelled. A major impetus for the discovery was the 1898 war between Spain and the United States over the ownership of Cuba. The Americans won, but for every soldier killed in battle 13 died from yellow fever. Cuba, in which the United States had strong economic interests in sugar production, was clearly a dangerous place. In response, Major William Gorgas was appointed the Chief Sanitary Officer in 1898 to tackle the yellow fever problem. Following the widely accepted miasma theory of disease, he initiated a clean-up programme to remove the filth from the cities of Cuba. Despite intensive efforts, deaths from yellow fever increased [14, 15].

In another initiative, an American research team of four doctors, led by Walter Reed, was sent to Cuba in 1900 to uncover the way the disease was spread. They quickly dismissed the miasma theory of corrupted air arising in dank humid places. With some reluctance they turned to the research undertaken by a Cuban doctor, Carlos Finlay. His work suggested that the disease was spread by mosquitoes, specifically one called *Aedes aegypti*. Walter Reed's team may also have been influenced by the investigations of Ronald Ross, a Scottish doctor working in India. He had shown in 1898 that malaria, another feared disease, was also spread by mosquitoes [14, 16, 17].

After reviewing all the evidence, the team decided to test if the mosquito theory could explain the spread of yellow fever. Two of the team doctors and a soldier volunteered to be bitten by an infected *Aedes aegypti* mosquito. All three developed yellow fever, but sadly one of the doctors, Jesse Lazear, died from the infection. Further studies identified how the infection was spread by mosquitoes. First, people with yellow fever can only pass the virus to biting mosquitoes during the early stages of their illness. The virus then has to incubate in the mosquito for about 2 weeks before it can be passed into humans. This process may seem an unlikely way to transmit an infection. But in the regions where yellow fever thrives, lots of people are being bitten frequently so the disease can spread. With crowded towns and cities, and untold thousands of mosquitoes, it can quickly cause a large outbreak. However, the important conclusion the research was that yellow fever could be prevented by killing mosquitoes. And the main target for extermination was the mosquito *Aedes aegypti* [14, 16, 17].

Cuba and the Panama Canal

The availability of a strategy to prevent outbreaks prompted the American military in 1901 to propose the elimination of the mosquito from the large towns and cities of Cuba. *Aedes aegypti* is adapted to feeding on humans, much preferring them to monkeys. It particularly likes an urban environment where it can breed in drinking water containers and any discarded items that can hold water. The person charged with controlling yellow fever, Major William Gorgas, implemented an extermination strategy as if it were a military campaign. To prevent person to mosquito to person spread, yellow fever victims were isolated. Their houses and the hospitals they visited were fumigated by burning sulphur or spraying with pyrethrum (both powerful insecticides). Gorgas sent out teams to drain the pools of pools water and to remove or cover containers that could catch rainwater. The result was that first Havana, and then the other major Cuban cities, were cleared of yellow fever [18–20].

The experience that Gorgas gained in Cuban proved invaluable for the building of the Panama Canal. It had been recognised for some time that a canal would provide a passage between the Pacific and Atlantic oceans, shortening the voyage from Southeast Asia to Europe by over 2000 miles. The work was begun, with much pomp, circumstance and champagne, by the French in 1881. Many challenges were encountered, in part because of poor planning for the engineering work. But the main hazard was illness and death. The region of Panama in which the canal was being built had a fearsome reputation. It was infested with yellow fever and malaria, making it one of the worst plague spots in the world. The exact scale of the mortality was not recorded, but it is thought that up to half of the men working on the canal died from infectious diseases. After spending $260 million, substantially more than was budgeted, the French abandoned the task in 1888. It sold all rights, and their engineering equipment, to the United States for $40 million [21, 22].

The Americans enthusiastically took on the task that the French had abandoned. They identified the engineering challenges and carefully planned how to overcome them. Maintaining a healthy workforce initially proved more difficult. Mortality was so high that many managers and engineers had brought funeral caskets with them so that their remains could be shipped home with some dignity. This changed when William Gorgas, now promoted to Colonel, was put in charge of preventing deaths from yellow fever and malaria by eliminating the mosquito. With dogged determination he overcame bureaucratic interference, lengthy delays and the ingrained view that the disease was spread by filth (miasma). His campaign used 300 tons of sulphur and 120 tons of pyrethrum, two effective insecticides, to fumigate dwellings. Some 600,000 gallons of oil were spread over ponds and swamps. This killed the mosquito larvae which live just under the surface of the water, by blocking the tubes that they used to breathe. Containers for water were fitted with fine wire gauze and piped water was introduced into houses to reduce reliance on water barrels. Many swamps were drained, and houses had screens fitted to exclude mosquitoes. As a result, yellow fever was eradicated in the Canal Zone and malaria infections were greatly reduced. The American success in building the Panama Canal owed much to the discovery of Walter Reed's team and the determination of William Gorgas [15, 21].

Expanding the Eradication Process

The successes in Cuba and Panama galvanised action to extend yellow fever eradication. Rio de Janeiro was the first to root out the disease in 1903. A workforce of 2500 men exterminated mosquitoes in 83,396 locations using the established techniques. Other cities—Santos (Brazil), Veracruz and Tampico (Mexico) and several urban centres in Panama—also succeeded in banishing the disease. By 1925 some countries, for example Ecuador, Peru, Colombia and Mexico, were free from the disease. These successes led to the belief that yellow fever outbreaks could be prevented by killing *Aedes aegypti* mosquitoes in urban centres [23–25].

This enthusiasm was dampened in 1928 when a new outbreak erupted in Rio de Janeiro, 25 years after yellow fever had been eradicated. Hundreds of people died. One reason for this outbreak was that control measures had been relaxed and the workers were transferred to other duties. But there was another more worrying explanation that emerged from a study of outbreaks in Brazil, Colombia and Venezuela. This suggested that there was another source of these new cases in the rainforests of tropical South America. Here the infection was maintained in a sylvatic (jungle) cycle from mosquitoes to monkeys to mosquitoes. It involved different species of mosquitoes (mainly species of the Haematosis and Sabethes genera) which are adapted to life in the rainforest. People living on the periphery of these rainforests are occasionally infected and can spread the disease to towns and cities where *Aedes aegypti* is common. Yellow fever spread rapidly in these urban environments. But why was yellow fever present in the rainforests? The answer lies in the origin of yellow fever, and in human greed and a marked insensitivity to the suffering others [19, 26] [27].

The Origin and Spread of Yellow Fever

Amidst all the efforts at controlling yellow fever, one question remained unresolved: where did the disease come from? Many people thought it had originated in the Americas, because the first recorded outbreak, and most of the subsequent ones, were in that region. But the true home was in the rainforests of equatorial Africa. The disease is caused by a virus that was descended from a strain of yellow fever that had circulated among non-human primates for hundreds of thousands years ago. It was maintained in a sylvatic (jungle) cycle from the mosquito *Aedes africanus* to apes and monkeys and then to mosquitoes [28]..

A novel strain of the virus emerged in West Africa about 3000 years ago. It spread widely among the *Aedes africanus* mosquitoes and in the non-human primates living in the rainforest. This virus strain was also good at infecting humans, so it was easily transmitted to those living in settlements on the edge of the rainforest. Possibly hunters seeking game in these forests were bitten by the *Aedes africanus* mosquitoes infected with this new strain. Or a jungle mosquito might have strayed into the hunter's village where there was a ready supply of human blood. These communities on the edge of the rainforest are described as zones of emergence. The *Aedes africanus* mosquitoes seed infections in zones of emergence, and the virus is then spread to towns and cities by the mosquito *Aedes aegypti*. This mosquito probably began specialising on humans as a source of blood meals about 5000 years ago. Having established itself in towns and cities, *Aedes aegypti* drives the urban cycle of infection with frequent transmission of yellow fever from mosquito to human and to mosquito [29, 30].

The first reported outbreak in Africa was among English troops stationed in Saint Louis, Senegal, in 1768. It initially affected men who had been ashore, then spread among those onboard. This is most likely just one of many outbreaks of yellow fever that have afflicted Africa over most of the last 1500 years. However, few records were kept until the 1920s when several large outbreaks were reported in Nigeria, Ghana and the Gambia. Initially it was thought that the disease was limited to a narrow strip of land on the West coast of Africa. Then it was realised that yellow fever was spread across equatorial Africa, from Senegal and Nigeria in the west to Kenya and Ethiopia in the east. Reports of large sporadic outbreaks began in the 1960s, and in the 1980s and 1990s Nigeria suffered several large outbreaks of thousands of cases. From the year 2000 onwards, moderate to large outbreaks have occurred across Africa. Possibly the largest ever outbreak in Africa hit Ethiopia from 1960 to 1963. An estimated 200,000 people were infected and about 30,000 died [31–34]..

The Spread to the Americas

From Africa yellow fever was transported to the Americas by the slave trade. The trade began in the 1400s when Europeans began exchanging trinkets, iron and cowrie shells for West African gold, ivory, pepper and slaves. The slaves were used to cultivate sugar cane, a high-value product, on the islands off the coast of North Africa. Columbus' discovery of the Americas in 1492, opened the way for traders and businessmen to expand the profitable Europe-West Africa system to include the Caribbean. The fertile soil and tropical climate of the Caribbean Islands were ideal for growing sugar cane on a large scale. All that was needed was a ready supply of slaves to do the work. At least 11 million native Africans were forcibly relocated from West Africa to the Americas from 1500 to 1850. The slaves were kept in appalling conditions, and many died, often from dehydration [35–37].

This slave trade, in which people were treated as commodities, not human beings, had an unexpected consequence. Not only did some of the slave ships carry people infected by yellow fever, they also carried the mosquito *Aedes aegypti*. There was a plentiful supply of these mosquitoes in coastal communities of West Africa. On board the ships there were humans to feed on and water containers for breeding. After arrival at the ports in the Americas, there was an even more plentiful supply of water containers and people for blood meals. It is not surprising that *Aedes aegypti* and the yellow fever virus flourished in this new environment.

There were a few outbreaks in the 1600s, but many more in the 1700s and 1800s. The frequency of yellow fever outbreaks in the Americas broadly corresponds to volume of slaves transported to that continent [9, 38, 39].

Seeding the Rainforest Reservoir

By far the most unfortunate consequence of the slave trade was the spread of the virus into the Amazonian rainforest. Here it was picked up by two different groups of mosquito (Haemogogous and Sabethes mosquitoes) which established mosquito to monkey to mosquito sylvatic cycles. This created a vast reservoir of yellow fever that could spill over into people living near to the rainforest. The human-adapted *Aedes aegypti* could then spread the virus to nearby communities and on to large towns and cities [9, 39].

The realisation that the tropical rainforest was the source of new outbreaks led to a new strategy targeted at the *Aedes aegypti* mosquito on the edges of the tropical rainforests. This was adopted in the 1930s by the Rockefeller foundation with the aim of preventing the infection from spreading to towns and cities. Brazil was chosen as a demonstration project, and the programme was such a success that by the 1940s it was almost entirely free from *Aedes aegypti*. This led to a 1947 resolution to mount elimination campaigns across the Americas. The availability of the new and highly effective insecticide DDT at the end of the Second World War greatly reduced the workload involved in killing mosquitoes. Progress was slower than expected, and, although many countries had successfully eliminated by the early 1970s, many others did not. What was particularly disappointing was that by the late 1970s the *Aedes aegypti* mosquito had spread to Brazil from neighbouring countries. It became widely distributed across Brazil which then suffered outbreaks of yellow fever in the early 1980s. In 1985 the countries of the Americas abandoned the aim of eradicating *Aedes aegypti* [40, 41].

Will It Spread to Asia?

A major concern is the potential for the spread of yellow fever to Asian countries such as India and China. The *Aedes aegypti* is widespread throughout this region, and laboratory studies have shown that the local strains of this mosquito are capable of spreading the yellow fever virus. Although several people infected with yellow fever have travelled to Asia, as yet there have been no cases of the disease that have been transmitted by local mosquitoes. For example during a large outbreak in Angola and the Democratic Republic of Congo in 2015–2016, 11 Chinese migrant workers became ill with yellow fever and returned home. Fortunately there was no onward spread of the infection. To ensure that yellow fever does not gain a foothold in Asia, WHO is seeking to enforce the International Health Regulations that require that anyone travelling from a yellow fever area has been vaccinated. If a major outbreak in Asia spread across the region, the consequences could be disastrous. Most people in Asia have no immunity to yellow fever [42–44].

The Vaccine

Towards the end of the nineteenth century, vaccines were increasingly seen as an effective method of preventing infectious diseases. Louis Pasteur made one of the key contributions by showing that a pathogenic microbe lost its virulence when repeatedly grown in a suitable culture medium. The early efforts to develop a yellow fever vaccine were based on the belief that the disease was caused by a bacterium. Several attempts were made, and one so-called bacterial vaccine was used extensively in the United States and Latin America. Then in 1927 Adrian Stokes, a professor of pathology, obtained blood from a patient named Asibi who had a mild form of yellow fever. From this sample Stokes was able to show that it was a virus, not a bacterium, that caused the disease. The supposed bacterial vaccine was quickly discarded, and efforts were directed at developing a vaccine against the yellow fever virus. The research was slow, painstaking and dangerous. Its first victim was Adrian Stokes himself who died from yellow fever shortly after he isolated the virus [45–47].

Following Louis Pasteur's lead, the first step was to weaken (attenuate) the virus by repeatedly passing it between mice. Then a simpler method used tissue from chicken embryos, with the virus being transferred from one tissue sample to the next for at least 100 times. These techniques were high risk. In 1931 some 32 US researchers from 8 laboratories became infected with yellow fever and 5 died. But in the early 1930s a prototype vaccine was developed by Max Theiler, a South African working in America. He used the virus that had been isolated from the patient Asibi. For his groundbreaking research he was awarded the Nobel Prize in 1951 [46, 47].

The main weakness of the early vaccine was that it sometimes caused unacceptable side effects. Many attempts were made to overcome this complication until, by chance, researchers stumbled upon a mutated version of the virus. After this strain of virus had been attenuated the resulting vaccine did not cause neurological side effects. The new vaccine was called 17D, and in 1937 it was produced on a large scale for use in population vaccination programmes. A highly effective vaccine with an excellent safety profile was now available for worldwide use. In the Americas in the 1930s and 1940s it was only used as an adjunct to *Aedes aegypti* eradication campaigns [40, 46, 47].

Using the same techniques as the US scientists, a French vaccine was developed by a team comprising two French and one American scientists working in the Pasteur Institute in Dakar, Senegal. This vaccine was also highly effective. It was given to patients by scarification—applying some liquid to skin that had been scratched. This technique meant the vaccine could be administered quickly, making it suitable for mass vaccination campaigns. Widely used in the French colonies in West Africa, an estimated 56 million people had been vaccinated by 1953. Where these campaigns were conducted, yellow fever became a rare disease. Because it caused rare neurological side effects, this vaccine was finally withdrawn in 1982 [47].

The new 17D vaccines arrived just in time to be used in the Second World War. Troops in North Africa were at risk of infection and mass vaccination campaigns were conducted, with 7 million doses being administered. Unfortunately, there were complications with over 25,000 soldiers developing jaundice. Some batches of vaccine had been contaminated with a hepatitis virus. To prevent this from happening again the production process was modified. Since then other adverse effects of the vaccine have been identified. Although most were mild and short term, some rare ones were more serious, such as anaphylaxis (a strong allergic reaction) and nerve damage. But the risk of side effects was much less than that of severe illness and death from the infection [47, 48].

Vaccination programmes in Africa and the Americas have had a major impact on infection rates. Based on the coverage achieved by 2016, about 100,000 cases of yellow fever were prevented each year. However, many of those living in yellow fever zones have not been vaccinated. Using data up to 2016 it is estimated that about 500 million people are at risk, with 90% of them living in Africa [49, 50].

Recent Outbreaks

Several large outbreaks of yellow fever have occurred of the past decade. One began in Angola in December 2015 and subsequently spread to the Democratic Republic of Congo. It continued until November 2016, causing an estimated 7300 cases and 393 deaths. Shortly after, Brazil experienced an outbreak that lasted from December 2016 to June 2019 and resulted in 2237 cases and 759 deaths. Then between 2017 and 2019 Nigeria suffered an outbreak that resulted in 7894 cases and 213 deaths. Africa is continuing to experience outbreaks [44, 51–53].

The EYE Strategy

In response to the Angola 2015/2016 outbreak, WHO and partners launched the EYE strategy (Eliminate Yellow fever Epidemics) in 2017. It was to be conducted over a 10-year period (2017–2026). The strategy had three main aims: to protect at risk populations, to prevent international spread and to contain outbreaks rapidly. The strategy focused on countries at high risk of yellow fever determined by their previous history of outbreaks, experience of conducting mass vaccination campaigns and recent history of infections. This identified 27 countries in Africa and a further 13 in Central and South America [54, 55].

Several actions were taken. Yellow fever vaccination was incorporated into the global programmes of routine immunisation of children. One long-term aim of this ensure was to ensure that in 30 years' time population immunity levels will be high (i.e. over 80%). A more immediate approach was to conduct mass vaccination campaigns in high-risk areas. In addition, vaccination was targeted at specific groups in the population who had low levels of immunity. Finally, improved surveillance will be used to detect yellow fever outbreaks in their early stages with rapid implementation of local vaccination programmes to reduce the spread of the virus [54].

The World Health Organization recommends that vaccinating 80% of the population would be sufficient to prevent outbreaks from spreading. For parts of West Africa and Equatorial Latin America where the risk of infection is particularly high, vaccination rates of 90% or even 95% may be needed. Substantial progress has been made. Recent estimates show that in South America many regions of Brazil, Bolivia and Paraguay are at or near the WHO 80% threshold, and that Colombia, Ecuador and Guyana have reached it for people aged less than 20. Some of the at-risk countries in Africa, such as Cameroon, Ghana, the Gambia and Senegal, are also near or have reached the 80% threshold. However, others are falling far short of that target (Ethiopia, Kenya, Mauritania Nigeria and South Sudan) [50, 56, 57].

The main problem with the vaccine is a shortage of supplies. The manufacturing process uses fertilised chicken eggs to grow the attenuated virus 17D. It takes about 5000 eggs to make one million doses of the vaccine. This limits the number of vaccines produced to between 33 and 80 million doses per year. WHO estimates that 1.38 billion doses of vaccine will be required over the period 2017–2026 to meet their targets. This equates to 138 million doses per year, leaving a shortfall of almost 60 million doses annually. But there is hope. The current vaccine is referred to as a legacy vaccine, as it still uses the techniques that were developed some 80 years ago. However recent research has established several new methods of producing vaccines, such as the mRNA technique that proved so effective against Covid 19. Although still in the early stages of testing, these candidate vaccines hold the promise that production of a low-cost vaccine can be scaled up to meet the global demand [57–59].

When Will it Will End?

Based on recent estimates there are about 109,000 cases and 51,000 deaths from yellow fever each year. Most of these, 92%, occur in Africa and the rest in South America. The top three countries in Africa are the Democratic Republic of Congo, Nigeria and Cameroon, although a dozen other countries have substantial amounts of the disease. Mass vaccination efforts in Africa reduced the number of deaths by an estimated 47%. In the Americas, Brazil stands out as having many more cases than all the other countries in that continent. This is not due to low vaccination coverage, but instead due to the intensity of mosquito biting [34].

The existence of large reservoirs of virus in the tropical rainforests of Africa and South America makes it unlikely that yellow fever can be eradicated. People living at the edge of the rainforests can be infected by jungle mosquitoes. This is the main source of outbreaks in sub-Saharan Africa. Widespread forest fragmentation also increases the risk of yellow fever outbreaks. Large areas of jungle are broken into smaller patches surrounded by roads, cultivated land and new housing communities. This greatly expands the opportunities for people to be exposed to jungle mosquitoes. It probably accounts for much of the increase in yellow fever infections that Brazil has experienced since the early 2000s [27, 29, 60, 61].

The current programmes to control yellow fever will reduce the present burden of disease. If sufficient supplies of vaccine become available, the reduction will be substantial and may finally achieve the WHO targets. However, reluctance to be vaccinated because of inadequate knowledge and fears about adverse effects, and difficulties in accessing vaccination centres, could reduce coverage below the threshold of 80%. Further, reinfection from tropical rainforests may thwart attempts to bring infection rates down to low levels. Yellow fever will pose an ongoing threat well beyond the WHO target date of 2026. The only certainty is that there will be new outbreaks of yellow fever for many years to come [60–62].

References

1. Vainio, J., & Cutts, F. (1998). *Yellow fever.* World Health Organization. https://iris.who.int/bitstream/handle/10665/64455/WHO_EPI_GEN_98.11.pdf?sequence=1&isAllowed=y
2. Leonard, J. (1989). Carlos Finlay's life and the death of yellow jack. *Bulletin of the Pan American Health Organization, 23*(4), 438–452.
3. Gould, E. A., & Solomon, T. (2008). Pathogenic flaviviruses. *Lancet, 371*(9611), 500–509.
4. Monath, T. P. (2001). Yellow fever: An update. *Lancet Infectious Diseases, 1*(1), 11–20.
5. Johansson, M. A., Vasconcelos, P. F., & Staples, J. E. (2014). The whole iceberg: Estimating the incidence of yellow fever virus infection from the number of severe cases. *Transactions of the Royal Society of Tropical Medicine and Hygiene, 108*(8), 482–487.
6. Kleinert, R. D. V., Montoya-Diaz, E., Khera, T., Welsch, K., Tegtmeyer, B., Hoehl, S., et al. (2019). Yellow fever: Integrating current knowledge with technological innovations to identify strategies for controlling a re-emerging virus. *Viruses, 11*(10), 960.
7. Blake, J. B. (1968). Yellow fever in eighteenth century America. *Bulletin of the New York Academy of Medicine, 44*(6), 673–686.
8. Prata, A. (2000). Yellow fever. *Memórias do Instituto Oswaldo Cruz, 95*, 183–187.
9. Patterson, K. D. (1992). Yellow fever epidemics and mortality in the United States, 1693-1905. *Social Science & Medicine (1982), 34*(8), 855–865.
10. Holbrook, M. R. (2017). Historical perspectives on flavivirus research. *Viruses, 9*, 5.
11. Jácome, R., Carrasco-Hernández, R., Campillo-Balderas, J. A., López-Vidal, Y., Lazcano, A., Wenzel, R. P., et al. (2019). A yellow flag on the horizon: The looming threat of yellow fever to North America. *International Journal of Infectious Diseases, 87*, 143–150.
12. Marr, J. S., & Cathey, J. T. (2013). The 1802 saint-Domingue yellow fever epidemic and the Louisiana purchase. *Journal of Public Health Management and Practice, 19*(1), 77–82.

13. Elman, C. (2004). Extending offensive realism: The Louisiana purchase and America's rise to regional hegemony. *American Political Science Review, 98*, 563–576.
14. Bryan, C. S., Moss, S. W., & Kahn, R. J. (2004). Yellow fever in the Americas. *Infectious Disease Clinics of North America, 18*(2), 275–292.
15. Gandy, R. E., Christopher, R. M., & Rodning, C. B. (2017). The statesmanship of William Crawford Gorgas, M.D., surgeon general, medical corps, United States army. *The American Surgeon, 83*(3), 221–232.
16. Reed, W., Carroll, J., & Agramonte, A. (2001). The etiology of yellow fever: An additional note. 1901. *Military Medical, 166*(9 Suppl), 44–53.
17. Clements, A. N., & Harbach, R. E. (2017). History of the discovery of the mode of transmission of yellow fever virus. *Journal of Vector Ecology, 42*(2), 208–222.
18. Webb, J. L., Jr. (2016). Aedes aegypti suppression in the Americas: Historical perspectives. *Lancet, 388*(10044), 556–557.
19. Camargo, S. (1967). History of Aedes aegypti eradication in the Americas. *Bulletin of the World Health Organization, 36*(4), 602–603.
20. Leonard, J. (1991). William Gorgas, soldier of public health. *Bulletin of the Pan American Health Organization, 25*(2), 166–185.
21. Orenstein, A. (1912). The sanitation of the canal zone. *Scientific American, 107*, 392–393.
22. Gorgas. (1914). Anti-mosquito work at Panama. *Proceedings of the Royal Society of Medicine, 7*, 31.1–40.1.
23. Camargo, S. (1971). *Vector control in urban areas.* World Health Organization.
24. Carrigan, J. (1988). Mass communication and public health: The 1905 campaign against yellow fever in New Orleans. *Journal of the Louisiana Historical Association, 29*, 5–20.
25. Soper, F. L. (1967). Aedes aegypti and yellow fever. *Bulletin of the World Health Organization, 36*(4), 521–527.
26. Soper, F. L. (1937). The newer epidemiology of yellow fever. *American Journal of Public Health and the Nation's Health, 27*(1), 1–14.
27. Li, S. L., Acosta, A. L., Hill, S. C., Brady, O. J., de Almeida, M. A. B., Cardoso, J. D. C., et al. (2022). Mapping environmental suitability of Haemagogus and Sabethes spp. mosquitoes to understand sylvatic transmission risk of yellow fever virus in Brazil. *PLoS Neglected Tropical Diseases, 16*(1), e0010019.
28. Barrett, A. D., & Higgs, S. (2007). Yellow fever: A disease that has yet to be conquered. *Annual Review of Entomology, 52*, 209–229.

29. Chippaux, J. P., & Chippaux, A. (2018). Yellow fever in Africa and the Americas: A historical and epidemiological perspective. *Journal of Venomous Animals and Toxins Including Tropical Diseases, 24*, 20.
30. Rose, N. H., Badolo, A., Sylla, M., Akorli, J., Otoo, S., Gloria-Soria, A., et al. (2023). Dating the origin and spread of specialization on human hosts in Aedes aegypti mosquitoes. *eLife*, 12, e83524.
31. Tomori, O. (2002). Yellow fever in Africa: Public health impact and prospects for control in the 21st century. *Biomédica, 22*(2), 178–210.
32. Findlay, G. M. (1941). The present position of yellow fever in Africa. *Transactions of the Royal Society of Tropical Medicine and Hygiene, 35*, 51–72.
33. Henderson, B. E., Metselaar, D., Cahill, K., Timms, G. L., Tukei, P. M., & Williams, M. C. (1968). Yellow fever immunity surveys in northern Uganda and Kenya and eastern Somalia, 1966-67. *Bulletin of the World Health Organization, 38*(2), 229–237.
34. Gaythorpe, K. A., Hamlet, A., Jean, K., Garkauskas Ramos, D., Cibrelus, L., Garske, T., et al. (2021). The global burden of yellow fever. *eLife, 10*, e64670.
35. Sheridan, R. B. (1972). Africa and the Caribbean in the Atlantic slave trade. *The American Historical Review, 77*, 15–35.
36. Maxwell, K. (1992). Portugal, Europe, and the origins of the Atlantic commercial system, 1415–1520. *Portugese Studies, 8*, 3–16.
37. Cohn, R. (1985). Deaths of slaves in the middle passage. *The Journal of Economic History, 45*, 685–692.
38. Johansson, M. A., Arana-Vizcarrondo, N., Biggerstaff, B. J., & Staples, J. E. (2010). Incubation periods of yellow fever virus. *The American Journal of Tropical Medicine and Hygiene, 83*(1), 183–188.
39. Silva, N. I. O., Albery, G. F., Arruda, M. S., Oliveira, G. F. G., Costa, T. A., de Mello, É. M., et al. (2023). Ecological drivers of sustained enzootic yellow fever virus transmission in Brazil, 2017-2021. *PLoS Neglected Tropical Diseases, 17*(6), e0011407.
40. Löwy, I. (2017). Leaking containers: Success and failure in controlling the mosquito aedes aegypti in Brazil. *American Journal of Public Health, 107*(4), 517–524.
41. Stepan, N. L. Could we/should we eradicate mosquitoes? The case of the yellow fever vector. In M. Hall & D. Tamïr (Eds.), *Mosquitopia: The place of pests in a healthy world* (pp. 73, 2022–86). Routledge.

42. Kuno, G. (2020). The absence of yellow fever in Asia: History, hypotheses, vector dispersal, possibility of YF in Asia, and other enigmas. *Viruses, 12*(12), 1349.
43. Gabiane, G., Yen, P. S., & Failloux, A. B. (2022). Aedes mosquitoes in the emerging threat of urban yellow fever transmission. *Reviews in Medical Virology, 32*(4), e2333.
44. Lindsey, N. P., Horton, J., Barrett, A. D. T., Demanou, M., Monath, T. P., Tomori, O., et al. (2022). Yellow fever resurgence: An avoidable crisis? *npj Vaccines, 7*(1), 137.
45. Payette, P. J., & Davis, H. L. (2001). History of vaccines and positioning of current trends. *Current Drug Targets. Infectious Disorders, 1*(3), 241–247.
46. Staples, J. E., & Monath, T. P. (2008). Yellow fever: 100 years of discovery. *Journal of the American Medical Association, 300*(8), 960–962.
47. Frierson, J. G. (2010). The yellow fever vaccine: A history. *The Yale Journal of Biology and Medicine, 83*(2), 77–85.
48. Lindsey, N. P., Schroeder, B. A., Miller, E. R., Braun, M. M., Hinckley, A. F., Marano, N., et al. (2008). Adverse event reports following yellow fever vaccination. *Vaccine, 26*(48), 6077–6082.
49. Shearer, F. M., Longbottom, J., Browne, A. J., Pigott, D. M., Brady, O. J., Kraemer, M. U. G., et al. (2018). Existing and potential infection risk zones of yellow fever worldwide: A modelling analysis. *The Lancet Global Health, 6*(3), e270–e278.
50. Shearer, F. M., Moyes, C. L., Pigott, D. M., Brady, O. J., Marinho, F., Deshpande, A., et al. (2017). Global yellow fever vaccination coverage from 1970 to 2016: An adjusted retrospective analysis. *The Lancet Infectious Diseases, 17*(11), 1209–1217.
51. Kraemer, M. U. G., Faria, N. R., Reiner, R. C., Jr., Golding, N., Nikolay, B., Stasse, S., et al. (2017). Spread of yellow fever virus outbreak in Angola and The Democratic Republic of the Congo 2015-16: A modelling study. *The Lancet Infectious Diseases, 17*(3), 330–338.
52. de Oliveira, F. P., Stoffella-Dutra, A. G., Barbosa Costa, G., Silva de Oliveira, J., Dourado Amaral, C., Duarte Santos, J., et al. (2020). Re-emergence of yellow fever in Brazil during 2016-2019: Challenges, lessons learned, and perspectives. *Viruses, 12*(11), 1233.
53. Nomhwange, T., Jean Baptiste, A. E., Ezebilo, O., Oteri, J., Olajide, L., Emelife, K., et al. (2021). The resurgence of yellow fever outbreaks in Nigeria: a 2-year review 2017-2019. *BMC Infectious Diseases, 21*(1), 1054.

54. World Health Organization. (2017). Eliminate yellow fever epidemics (EYE): A global strategy, 2017–2026. *Weekly Epidemiological Record, 92*(16), 193–204.
55. Anonymous. (2017). Eliminate yellow fever epidemics (EYE): A global strategy, 2017–2026. *Weekly Epidemiological Record, 92*(16), 193–204.
56. Ndeffo-Mbah, M. L., & Pandey, A. (2020). Global risk and elimination of yellow fever epidemics. *The Journal of Infectious Diseases, 221*(12), 2026–2034.
57. Hansen, C. A., & Barrett, A. D. T. (2021). The present and future of yellow fever vaccines. *Pharmaceuticals (Basel), 14*(9), 891.
58. Zurbia-Flores, G., Rollier, C., & Reyes-Sandoval, A. (2022). Re-thinking yellow fever vaccines: Fighting old foes with new generation vaccines. *Human Vaccines & Immunotherapeutics, 18*(1), 1895644.
59. Medina-Magües, L., Mühe, J., Jasny, E., et al. (2023). Immunogenicity and protective activity of mRNA vaccine candidates against yellow fever virus in animal models. *npj Vaccines, 8*(1), 31.
60. Uchenna Emeribe, A., Nasir Abdullahi, I., Ajagbe, O. O. R., Egede Ugwu, C., Oloche Onoja, S., Dahiru Abubakar, S., et al. (2021). Incidence, drivers and global health implications of the 2019/2020 yellow fever sporadic outbreaks in sub-Saharan Africa. *Pathogens and Disease, 79*(4), ftab017.
61. Rosser, J. I., Nielsen-Saines, K., Saad, E., & Fuller, T. (2022). Reemergence of yellow fever virus in southeastern Brazil, 2017-2018: What sparked the spread? *PLoS Neglected Tropical Diseases, 16*(2), e0010133.
62. Lopes, V. D. S., Souza, P. C., Garcia, É. M., & Lima, J. C. (2023). Yellow fever vaccine hesitancy and its relationship with contextual, individual, or group influences and vaccine-specific issues: A scoping review. *Ciência & Saúde Coletiva, 28*(6), 1717–1727.

Leprosy

Leprosy is a physically, psychologically and socially destructive disease. The initial signs of infection are pale or reddish spots which increase in size and become raised. The term 'leprosy' derives from the Greek word *léprā*, describing the scaly appearance of the skin. Infection causes damage to the nerves in the skin. This makes the affected areas numb, although sometimes they can have tingling or burning sensations. As the disease progresses, the face, upper and lower limbs can be covered in lumps (nodules), eyelashes and eyebrows can fall out and patients lose the ability to blink. The tissues in the nose can be attacked, leading to the collapse of the bridge of the nose, a condition called saddle-nose deformity. Muscles in the hands and feet may become paralysed so that the victims are crippled. A common example is the 'claw hand', in which fingers become fixed in a curved position resembling a bear's claw. Loss of sensation in the skin means that patients suffer repeated trauma which leads to bacterial or fungal infections. Inflammation in the eyes can lead to blindness. With modern antibiotic treatment the disease can be cured, although lesions on damaged skin can persist for several years [1–3].

The disease is mainly caused by the bacterium *Mycobacterium leprae* (*M. leprae*). (A few cases result from infection with another bacterium, *M. lepromatosis*.) The severity of infection varies. In mild disease, often

© The Author(s), under exclusive license to Springer Nature Singapore Pte Ltd. 2025
I. K Crombie, *Major Pandemics*, https://doi.org/10.1007/978-981-95-2081-7_5

termed paucibacillary or tuberculoid leprosy, patients harbour less than one million bacteria. They have only a few, localised and well-defined skin lesions and limited nerve damage. In contrast, *patients with* severe *disease (multibacillary or lepromatous) can host up to 100 billion bacteria. This high concentration of bacteria causes trauma to* the skin, the peripheral nerves and the cells lining the upper respiratory tract leading to disfiguring severe disease [2, 4, 5].

Stigmatisation in History and Religion

The disfigurement and deformities of leprosy place a heavy burden on those with this disease: it 'destroys not only the body but the soul'. Possibly even worse is the stigma and discrimination that people with leprosy have to confront. Repugnance and fear are common responses to the sight of a leper, with rejection and social exclusion as the consequence. Some misplaced beliefs have exacerbated the adverse effect of stigma. The book of Leviticus in the Old Testament presented leprosy as a plague sent by God to punish those who do not follow the spiritual and social rules of behaviour. They were deemed unclean and were to be excluded from society to prevent moral or physical contamination. The original Hebrew term used, *zaraat* or *şâra'ath*, refers to a variety of skin diseases rather than a specific disease. Unfortunately, it was translated as leprosy, although this disease was probably not present in biblical times [6, 7].

In the Middle Ages, communities across Europe had mixed views on leprosy. Some regarded the victims as untrustworthy, unclean and suspicious. They were often accused of poisoning wells or were blamed for economic and social misfortunes. Being judged unclean, they could be forbidden to enter churches, markets and inns. In some places they had to carry a bell or a clapper to warn people that they were coming. Many were often forced to live in separate encampments. However, other communities took a more compassionate approach, allowing those with leprosy to travel freely, visit markets and even own property. They could also be housed in leprosaria (specially built hospices or hospitals) buildings which provided safety and support in what was at times a hostile world [8, 9].

Some Hindus believe that the disease is inflicted upon people for sinful and immoral behaviour in a previous life. They were often socially excluded. However, if treated and cured the sufferer could be readmitted to society. In general Moslems have a more tolerant attitude to leprosy: 'Allah does not look at your outward form and your bodies, but he looks at your heart and your deeds'. Their sacred texts deal with how to be protected from leprosy while helping those who suffer from it. The teachings of the Buddha also take a supportive approach to disease encapsulated in the phrase 'whoever serves the sick serves me'. Overall, the history of leprosy is one where some peoples and communities were supportive of lepers while others shunned them. Stigma and discrimination remain a serious problem today [10–12].

Origin and Spread

Leprosy is thought to have infected humans for thousands of years, although where it originated and the routes of its spread are unclear. Evidence of bone malformations consistent with leprosy has been identified in skeletons from Hungary about 3700 BCE and in India from 2000 BCE. Historical texts provide tantalising accounts of where and when the disease may have been present, without shedding light on its origin. Egyptian papyri from 1550 BCE describe a disease that could be leprosy, as do religious texts from India about 1400 BCE. None of these early sources provide conclusive evidence of leprosy. More convincing is an ancient Sanskrit medical text from India (600 BCE). In Europe the first reliable case descriptions come from the medical texts of ancient Greece about 150 CE [13–15].

Studies on bacterial DNA in skeletons from ancient cemeteries provide some clues of the origins of leprosy, although the available evidence has been described as 'fragmentary, ambiguous and sometimes contradictory'. Recent findings suggest that the leprosy bacterium diverged from a common ancestor 13.9 million years ago, although the *M. leprae* that we know today first emerged somewhere between 5500 and 2000 years ago. At one time it was thought that India was the likely place of origin of leprosy. Then more recent studies suggest that it had originated in East

Africa or the Middle East. Other possible candidates include China and Myanmar. Until more evidence from ancient DNA is unearthed, the present position is one of speculation rather than firm conclusions [2, 13, 16].

Early Spread

Four major strains of leprosy have been identified, types 1–4, and these have enabled researchers to begin to map the global spread of leprosy. However, the early spread of leprosy is steeped in as much uncertainty as the evidence for its origin. In the remote past, more than 40,000 years ago, leprosy could have been spread by human migration, as groups of people moved to find better lives in new areas. One suggestion is that the disease spread from East Africa or the Eastern Mediterranean all the way to China. It may have followed two different routes. The southern one involved both land and sea travel, progressed through southern India and then to China. The northern route followed the Silk Road through Turkey and Iran and across central Asia to China [2, 16–18].

A less plausible explanation is that the disease first emerged in India and was carried back to Europe by the soldiers of Alexander the Great in 326 BCE. This is unlikely because the strains of leprosy in Europe (mainly type 3 and type 2) are largely different from those that circulated in India (mainly type 1). Another questionable suggestion is that, following a successful campaign in Anatolia in 62 BCE, the troops of the Roman general Pompey could have introduced the disease to Italy. What is clear is that leprosy was present in some of the southern European countries in the first few centuries CE. It is likely that as the Roman legions progressively conquered Western Europe, they also spread leprosy throughout the region. Because there are so few reports of outbreaks during the Roman period, the disease may have been either mild or only slightly infectious [13, 19, 20].

The nature of leprosy infection changed about 500 CE when people from Central and East Asia migrated westwards in a series of waves. At some stage they may have introduced new strains of leprosy into Western Europe. This may explain why the disease had become much more common by 1000 CE. It stayed that way for the next 300 years. Over that time many leper-houses and hospitals, often associated with monasteries, were built across the region. After 1300 CE the frequency of infection progressively fell until the disease had largely disappeared by the seventeenth century. There has been much speculation about the reasons for the progressive reduction in cases across most of Western Europe. Enforced segregation of people in leper-houses and hospitals is thought to provide part of the explanation. But it is more likely that improvements in standards of living such as less overcrowding and better nutrition were the major factors [15, 18].

Across the Atlantic

Leprosy was spread by Europeans to West Africa and the Americas. This probably occurred in a series of waves that started in the late Middle Ages, with the slave trade playing the major role. European ships raided coastal West Africa capturing the local inhabitants and transporting them to the Caribbean Islands and mainland North and South America. There they were forced to work, initially on sugar-cane plantations. Through a combination of hard labour, poor nutrition and crowded conditions, infectious diseases, including leprosy, were rife. When current ones died from these diseases, new slaves were bought because that was cheaper than providing decent living conditions [21, 22].

As is the way with infectious diseases, leprosy quickly spread into local communities. Many of the Caribbean Islands and countries in South America, such as Brazil, Paraguay, Colombia, Argentina and Venezuela, suffered from this proliferation of the disease. One long-term consequence is that Brazil currently has the second highest number of new cases of leprosy in the world. In the southern United States, leprosy was transmitted by slaves, and by other peoples, such as those of Spanish descent and French-speaking Acadians. Texas, Florida and Louisiana were noted as centres of infection up to the twentieth century. The disease had been present in most other states at one time or other, but three stand out: California, New York and Hawaii. All had substantial numbers of immigrants who were the source of infection. Although leprosy has now virtually disappeared from the United States, recent evidence suggests that there is an ongoing trickle of new cases [23–25].

Finding the Cause

Although the frequency of leprosy in most of Western Europe was low from the seventeenth century onwards, the Scandinavian countries were different. Here the infection rumbled on until the number of cases began to increase from the end of the eighteenth century to the mid-nineteenth century. Norway experienced a particularly large increase in disease frequency over this time, and this encouraged research into the causes of leprosy. In 1849 a new research facility was established at the St Jørgen Hospital under the leadership of Dr. Daniel Danielssen. At that time leprosy was generally thought to be a hereditary disease, although a few doctors thought it might be contagious. In an effort to confirm that the disease was not passed from person to person, Danielssen and his co-workers inoculated each other with samples from patients with leprosy. Despite repeated attempts to transmit leprosy, no one succumbed to the disease [26, 27].

These findings, and others, supported the view that leprosy was a hereditary disease. It led to the suggestion that, in order to reduce the number of new cases, people with leprosy should not be allowed to have sexual intercourse. Another proposal was that all female patients with leprosy should be isolated and the male patients should be sterilised. Fortunately, none of these was put into action. Instead, a national register of leprosy patients in Norway was created to monitor trends in the disease and to support research into the causes of leprosy [26, 27].

Then in 1868 a young Norwegian doctor/researcher, Gerhard Henrik Armauer Hansen, began working at the St Jørgen Hospital. He became a trusted disciple of Dr. Danielssen. But research findings from Dutch Guiana (modern Suriname) inspired him to follow a different path. These showed that European settlers became infected only after living for several years in the new country. The conclusion was that leprosy might be infectious. To test this, Hansen investigated many family groups in Norway and found that only those individuals who had contact with a leprosy patient became infected with the disease. He also noted that when new leprosy hospitals were opened the number of new cases in the surrounding communities gradually declined. This suggested that the isolation of cases reduced the spread of disease. Finally, Hansen investigated fluids taken from patients with leprosy and identified rod-shaped particles that he thought could be the culprit bacterium. But demonstrating that these particles caused leprosy turned out to be difficult. Hansen was unable to cause the disease in experimental animals by injecting them with fluids from leprosy patients. Being able to pass infection from one animal to another was recognised as an essential requirement for showing that the particles were infectious [28, 29].

In an effort to confirm that leprosy was contagious, Hansen conducted an unethical study on a woman with a form of leprosy that causes severe sensory loss. Some fluid taken from another patient was inserted into the lady's eye. He reasoned that if the rod-shaped particles could multiply in a live human, they were probably the bacteria that caused the disease. Unfortunately, Hansen neglected to obtain informed consent before carrying out the procedure. He was prosecuted for this illegal action and dismissed from his post at Bergen Leprosy Hospital. Despite the disgrace that hung over Hansen, his achievements were gradually recognised and in 1897 the First International Congress of Leprology declared that leprosy was an infectious disease. The rod-shaped particles that Hansen had seen were accepted as the cause of leprosy and were given the scientific name *Mycobacterium leprae* (*M. leprae*). Possibly in recognition of Hansen's rehabilitation, but also to replace the stigmatising term 'leprosy', the 1931 International Leprosy Congress recommended renaming the disease. It was to be called Hansen's disease, in honour of the man who discovered the bacterium that causes it [29–31].

The confirmation that leprosy was contagious had an unfortunate consequence. Many countries introduced isolation as a means of reducing the spread of leprosy. This view was validated by the First International Congress on Leprosy in 1897 which concluded that as leprosy was incurable, compulsory isolation of leprosy patients was the best way to control the disease. This led to the construction of leprosaria which isolated the victims of this disease from society, their family and friends. It was not until 25 years later that humane segregation was gradually accepted as a better approach, providing comfortable surroundings and easy access to family members [32–34].

Infection by *M. leprae*

M. leprae invades a particular type of cell, the Schwann cell. It provides a coating for the nerves that send signals round the body, increasing the speed at which messages are sent. This cell also provides nutrients for the nerves. Only the Schwann cells in the skin are invaded because they are at a lower temperature than the rest of the body. The bacterium grows best in cooler places. Infection results in a loss of sensation in the skin because the nerves can no longer send signals. This leads to muscle atrophy and some bone loss [35, 36].

During its evolution *M. leprae* lost or inactivated about half of its genes. To compensate, it hijacks the biochemical machinery of the Schwann cell to provide the missing functions. This process may be the way the bacterium evolved to thrive in the foreign environment of human cells. It may also explain why *M. leprae* grows so much more slowly than most other bacteria [35, 36].

The Transmission of Leprosy

Despite substantial research, the details of person-to-person leprosy transmission are not fully understood. Part of the problem is that there is a long interval between the initial infection and the appearance of symptoms. The average period is about 5 years, although it can range from 2 to 12 years. This makes it difficult to determine the characteristics of the exposure that led to disease. That said, the main method of spread is thought to be by the coughs and sneezes of an existing case. This aerosol route is plausible because high concentrations of the bacterium are found in nasal discharges among patients with multibacilliary leprosy. A possible additional route is through direct physical contact with cuts and abrasions in the skin. There are several reports of leprosy lesions developing at the sites of tattooing, vaccinations and traumatic injury [37–39].

Extended periods of close proximity to an infected individual is the major risk factor for leprosy transmission. Among married couples the frequency of transfer from an infected spouse to the uninfected one is low, occurring in 3–5% of cases. This low rate of transmission occurs because most people have a natural genetic immunity to leprosy. Researchers have identified many human genes that contribute to susceptibility to infection and to the subsequent severity of disease. The risk of infection is higher among close relatives of the infected person such as children living in the same house. That is because the children receive half of their genes from the infected parent and will have some or possibly all of those that make them susceptible to disease [40, 41].

As with many infectious diseases, poverty increases the risk of succumbing to leprosy. Even within poor communities, the most deprived individuals are at a higher risk of being infected. Poverty may exert its effects through increased exposure due to overcrowding or to greater susceptibility because of sustained poor diet. Other risk factors associated with the risk of infection include older age, limited education and manual labour [42–44].

Leprosy can be contracted from animals such as the armadillo. In North America the nine-banded armadillo provides a natural reservoir of leprosy. In some regions of the United States as many as 20% of armadillos are infected with leprosy. They are now recognised as a source of human infection in the United States The six-banded armadillos in Brazil, which are hunted and reared for food, are also infected with leprosy. Those who handle armadillos, and butcher or eat their meat, are at risk of being infected with leprosy. It is not known whether the armadillo initially transmitted the disease to humans or whether it came from humans [2, 38, 45, 46].

Some of the red squirrels in Britain are infected with *M. leprae*. The use of squirrel fur on clothes was popular in the Late Middle Ages, so it is possible that cases of human leprosy were caused by dead squirrels hung around the necks of fine ladies and gentlemen. In modern times there is no evidence that red squirrels have passed the disease to humans, possibly because these shy animals keep well away from humans [47].

Treatment and Prevention

For most of its history, leprosy was seen as a disease without hope. But in the early 1950s a new antibiotic, dapsone, looked set to transform lives. It was effective, inexpensive and simple to administer, although it had to be taken every week for 5–10 years. Then problems emerged: the drug could sometimes be toxic, many patients were not cured and *M. leprae* was developing resistance to the drug. However, researchers had been seeking out alternative treatments and in the 1980s a multidrug treatment inspired new hope. The combination of rifampicin, clofazimine and dapsone was highly effective and had to be taken for a much shorter period, 6 months for mild leprosy and 12 months for severe disease. This combination of drugs was much less likely to lead to drug resistance. Uptake of the new treatment among diagnosed patients rose quickly from 1% in 1985 to 100% in 1997. The use of the multidrug therapy was greatly facilitated when first the Nippon Foundation, then the pharmaceutical company Novartis, provided funding so that every case in the world would receive free treatment. This was a triumph of collaboration between pharmaceutical companies, non-profit organisations, national governments and international agencies [48–50].

Although multidrug therapy is highly effective, delayed treatment of leprosy is a major problem. It can lead to disabilities such as visual impairment, claw hand and foot drop. Several factors combine to prevent the early treatment that could prevent these conditions. At the individual level, reluctance to seek care, particularly in the early stages of the disease, difficulties of access to care and perceived stigma are major barriers. Within the health system, the main problem is the delay in making the diagnosis of leprosy, possibly because of inadequate training [51–53].

As well as treating infected patients, one drug (rifampin) has been shown to be effective at protecting individuals recently exposed to a person with leprosy. This eliminates the bacterium in the very early stages of the infection. The level of protection is modest and is greater in people who live close to the infected person. This use of post-exposure prophylaxis could provide a method of reducing the number of new cases of leprosy [54, 55].

Global use of an effective vaccine provides another way to prevent the spread of leprosy. An early finding was that the BCG vaccine for tuberculosis (TB) was also effective against leprosy. The two bacteria *Mycobacterium tuberculosis* and *M. leprae* are closely related, so it is not surprising that the TB vaccine also had an effect on leprosy. The level of protection against leprosy varied substantially between countries, from 18% to 90%. The reasons for this variability are not well understood. However, using the vaccine in combination with post-exposure prophylaxis with rifampin has a greater effect than either on its own. Research on novel vaccines is an active field, and a more effective vaccine might become available in the next few years [56, 57].

Impact of the New Treatments

As the multidrug therapy became widely used, the number of newly registered cases fell rapidly from 5.4 million in 1985 to 1.3 million in 1995. By the year 2000 the global number had fallen to 752,000. It continued to fall to about 200,000 in 2014 and then stayed largely constant to 2019 [58, 59].

There is a puzzling feature in the trend of new cases after 2000. From a peak of 752,000 in 2000, the number fell to just under 300,000 cases in 2005. It seems biologically implausible for the new cases to fall so rapidly in such a short period of time. In the following 14 years, from 2006 to 2019, new cases fell by only 100,000. The most likely explanation is that it was an unintended consequence of a decision by the World Health Organization. It set a target of reducing the number of new and existing cases (expressed as a rate per 10,000 population) to less than 1 per 10,000. When this was achieved in the year 2000, WHO announced that leprosy had been eliminated. This may have encouraged many countries to transfer resources to other healthcare problems, leading to a reduction in case finding activities in the years following 2000. If true, many hundreds of thousands of cases will have been overlooked. Smith and colleagues referred to them as 'the missing millions'. These cases could represent a vast reservoir from which the infection could spread [60–63].

After 2019, the numbers detected become unreliable for a few years because the Covid-19 pandemic disrupted the identification of new cases. There appeared to be a rapid fall to about 130,000 in 2020, then a recovery to 174,000 in 2022 and to 182,800 a year later. The main point is that there has been little progress in controlling leprosy infections; from 2014 to 2023 the number of new cases only fell from 200,000 to 182,000 [25, 59].

Current Position

Leprosy is present in most countries of the world; only 54 of the 182 countries which supply data are free from the disease. Three countries accounted for 80% of the 182,000 new cases reported in 2023: India (59%), Brazil (13%) and Indonesia (8%). But several other countries reported having more than 2000 cases: Bangladesh, Democratic Republic of Congo, Ethiopia, Nepal and Nigeria. It is clear that the disease is predominant in South and Southeast Asia, with Africa and South America also contributing many cases [59].

As well as the frequency and global distribution of the disease, the impact of the disease is a major concern. Most of the new cases (69%) have the most serious form of the disease, multibacillary leprosy. Further, almost 10,000 of these cases presented with visible disabilities, indicating that there was a long interval between initial symptoms and diagnosis. In addition, over 13,000 of the cases had received treatment previously and were returning for further treatment after a period of absence. It is clear that improvements in early detection and methods to encourage patients to complete treatment are needed. Possibly the most tragic figure is that over 10,000 children were newly diagnosed with leprosy in 2023 [25, 59].

A worrying feature of leprosy is the growing evidence of hidden cases. Several recent and detailed investigations in high-burden countries have found that many cases were previously undetected. Concerns about stigma are the main cause of delayed case identification, although severe disease, lack of knowledge and poverty also contribute. Active case detection by tracing contacts of leprosy patients, house-to-house visits and prison visits can identify many new cases. But it is very resource-intensive, raising the question of priorities: how much funding should countries devote to leprosy and how much to diseases such as AIDS, tuberculosis and malaria [64–68].

When Will it End?

Efforts to tackle leprosy have made good progress, with 18 million people successfully treated so far. Given the high level of international commitment, and recent advances in leprosy control, could further improvements be made? In answer the World Health Organization launched its campaign Towards Zero Leprosy in 2021. This set ambitious aims for 2030. These are to have: at least 120 countries with no person-to-person spread; a reduction in the number of new cases by 70%; a reduction of 90% in the frequency of grade 2 disability and a 90% reduction in the number of new cases among children [69].

The impact of Covid-19 on the reporting of leprosy makes it is difficult to know what progress has been made towards the 2030 Zero Leprosy targets. The year 2030 may show that the targets have been met. Alternatively, the hidden cases could continue to spread the disease, keeping the number of new cases higher than would be wished. The experience of eradicating smallpox and the continuing efforts to do so for polio are that the final stages of disease control are the hardest to achieve. Leprosy may well remain a problem for many years to come [59, 70–72].

References

1. Yousaf, K. S. (2022). The etymology of microbial nomenclature and the diseases these cause in a historical perspective. *Saudi Journal of Biological Sciences, 29*(11), 103454.
2. Avanzi, C., Singh, P., Truman, R. W., & Suffys, P. N. (2020). Molecular epidemiology of leprosy: An update. *Infection, Genetics and Evolution, 86*, 104581.

3. Menger, D. J., Fokkens, W. J., Lohuis, P. J., Ingels, K. J., & Nolst Trenité, G. J. (2007). Reconstructive surgery of the leprosy nose: a new approach. *Journal of Plastic, Reconstructive & Aesthetic Surgery, 60*(2), 152–162.
4. Leprosy, D. D. (2004). In C. Murray, A. Lopez, & C. Mathers (Eds.), *The global epidemiology of infectious diseases. Global burden of disease and injury series. IV* (pp. 201–218). World Health Organization.
5. Serrano-Coll, H., Wan, E. L., Restrepo-Rivera, L., & Cardona-Castro, N. (2024). Leprosy reactions: Unraveling immunological mechanisms underlying tissue damage in leprosy patients. *Pathogens and Disease, 82*, ftae013.
6. Bainson, K. A., & Van den Borne, B. (1998). Dimensions and process of stigmatization in leprosy. *Leprosy Review, 69*(4), 341–350.
7. Grzybowski, A., & Nita, M. (2016). Leprosy in the Bible. *Clinics in Dermatology, 34*(1), 3–7.
8. Covey, H. (2001). People with leprosy (Hansen's disease) during the middle ages. *The Social Science Journal, 38*, 315–321.
9. Miller, T., & Smith-Savage, R. (2006). Medieval leprosy reconsidered. *International Social Science Review, 81*, 16–28.
10. Hasnain, R., Queijo, J., Suheil, L., et al. (2020). Islam, leprosy, and disability: How religion, history, art, and storytelling can yield new insights and acceptance. *Societies, 10*, 1–17.
11. Sermrittirong, S., & Van Brakel, W. H. (2014). Stigma in leprosy: Concepts, causes and determinants. *Leprosy Review, 85*(1), 36–47.
12. Raju, S., Rao, P., & Karthikeyan, G. (2020). Socio-medical perspectives on leprosy in Indian religions. *Leprosy Review, 91*, 190–199.
13. Strahorn, E. A. (2020). Reconsidering the early history of leprosy in light of advances in palaeopathology. In G. Campbell & E.-M. Knoll (Eds.), *Disease dispersion and impact in the Indian ocean world* (pp. 85–103). Springer International Publishing.
14. Trautman, J. R. (1984). A brief history of Hansen's disease. *Bulletin of the New York Academy of Medicine, 60*(7), 689–695.
15. Browne, S. G. (1975). Some aspects of the history of leprosy: The leprosie of yesterday. *Proceedings of the Royal Society of Medicine, 68*(8), 485–493.
16. Mark, S. (2019). The origin and spread of leprosy: Historical, skeletal, and molecular data. *Journal of Interdisciplinary History, 49*(3), 367–395.
17. Monot, M., Honoré, N., Garnier, T., Araoz, R., Coppée, J. Y., Lacroix, C., et al. (2005). On the origin of leprosy. *Science, 308*(5724), 1040–1042.

18. Donoghue, H. D., Michael Taylor, G., Marcsik, A., Molnár, E., Pálfi, G., Pap, I., et al. (2015). A migration-driven model for the historical spread of leprosy in medieval eastern and Central Europe. *Infection, Genetics and Evolution, 31*, 250–256.
19. Mark, S. (2002). Alexander the great, seafaring, and the spread of leprosy. *Journal of the History of Medicine and Allied Sciences, 57*(3), 285–311.
20. Pfrengle, S., Neukamm, J., Guellil, M., Keller, M., Molak, M., Avanzi, C., et al. (2021). Mycobacterium leprae diversity and population dynamics in medieval Europe from novel ancient genomes. *BMC Biology, 19*(1), 220.
21. Block, K. (2017). Slavery and inter-imperial leprosy discourse in the Atlantic world. *Atlantic Studies, 14*, 243–262.
22. Shuler, K. (2011). Life and death on a barbadian sugar plantation: Historic and bioarchaeological views of infection and mortality at Newton plantation. *International Journal of Osteoarchaeology, 21*, 66–81.
23. Munro, W. (1876). On the etiology and history of leprosy. *Edinburgh Medical Journal, 22*(3), 242–249.
24. Hudson, T., & Genesse, J. (1982). Hansen's disease in the United States. *Social Science & Medicine, 16*, 997–1004.
25. World Health Organisation. (2023). Global leprosy (Hansen disease) update, 2022: New paradigm—control to elimination. *Weekly Epidemiological Record, 98*(37), 409–430.
26. Irgens, L. (2010). The fight against leprosy in Norway in the 19th century. *Michael, 7*, 307–320.
27. Rees, R. J. (1973). A century of progress in experimental leprosy. *International Journal of Leprosy and Other Mycobacterial Diseases, 41*(3), 320–328.
28. Harboe, M. (1973). Armauer Hansen--the man and his work. *International Journal of Leprosy and Other Mycobacterial Diseases, 41*(4), 417–424.
29. Grybowski, A., Sak, J., Pawlikowski, J., et al. (2013). Gerhard Henrik Armauer Hansen (1841-1912)—The 100th anniversary of the death of the discoverer of mycobacterium leprae. *Clinics in Dermatology, 31*, 653–655.
30. Vogelsang, T. M. (1963). A serious sentence passed against the discoverer of the leprosy bacillus (Gerhard Armauer HANSEN), in 1880. *Medical History, 7*(2), 182–186.
31. Deps, P., & Cruz, A. (2020). Why we should stop using the word leprosy. *The Lancet Infectious Diseases, 20*(4), e75–ee8.
32. Gussow, Z., & Tracy, G. S. (1970). Stigma and the leprosy phenomenon: The social history of a disease in the nineteenth and twentieth centuries. *Bulletin of the History of Medicine, 44*(5), 425–449.

33. Sato, H., & Frantz, J. E. (2005). Termination of the leprosy isolation policy in the US and Japan: Science, policy changes, and the garbage can model. *BMC International Health and Human Rights, 5*(1), 3.
34. Jing, L., & Long, L. (2017). The dawn of humane leprosy segregation: Transforming leprosarium into home. *International Journal of Sustainable Built Environment, 4*, 1–9.
35. Hess, S., & Rambukkana, A. (2019). Cell biology of intracellular adaptation of mycobacterium leprae in the peripheral nervous system. *Microbiology Spectrum, 7*(4), 20.
36. Chavarro-Portillo, B., Soto, C. Y., & Guerrero, M. I. (2019). Mycobacterium leprae's evolution and environmental adaptation. *Acta Tropica, 197*, 105041.
37. Schreuder, P. A., Noto, S., & Richardus, J. H. (2016). Epidemiologic trends of leprosy for the 21st century. *Clinics in Dermatology, 34*(1), 24–31.
38. Ploemacher, T., Faber, W. R., Menke, H., Rutten, V., & Pieters, T. (2020). Reservoirs and transmission routes of leprosy; a systematic review. *PLoS Neglected Tropical Diseases, 14*(4), e0008276.
39. Ghorpade, A. (2009). Post-traumatic inoculation tuberculoid leprosy after injury with a glass bangle. *Leprosy Review, 80*(2), 215–218.
40. Joyce, M. P. (2012). Historic aspects of human susceptibility to leprosy and the risk of conjugal transmission. *Memórias do Instituto Oswaldo Cruz, 107*(Suppl 1), 17–21.
41. Fava, V. M., Dallmann-Sauer, M., & Schurr, E. (2020). Genetics of leprosy: Today and beyond. *Human Genetics, 139*(6–7), 835–846.
42. Nery, J. S., Ramond, A., Pescarini, J. M., Alves, A., Strina, A., Ichihara, M. Y., et al. (2019). Socioeconomic determinants of leprosy new case detection in the 100 million Brazilian cohort: A population-based linkage study. *The Lancet Global Health, 7*(9), e1226–e1e36.
43. Pescarini, J. M., Strina, A., Nery, J. S., Skalinski, L. M., Andrade, K. V. F., Penna, M. L. F., et al. (2018). Socioeconomic risk markers of leprosy in high-burden countries: A systematic review and meta-analysis. *PLoS Neglected Tropical Diseases, 12*(7), e0006622.
44. Oktaria, S., Hurif, N. S., Naim, W., Thio, H. B., Nijsten, T. E. C., & Richardus, J. H. (2018). Dietary diversity and poverty as risk factors for leprosy in Indonesia: A case-control study. *PLoS Neglected Tropical Diseases, 12*(3), e0006317.
45. da Silva, F. J., de Carvalho, F. M., Vidal Pessolani, M. C., de Paula Antunes, J. M. A., de Medeiros Oliveira, I. V. P., Ferreira Moura, G. H., et al. (2020). Serological and molecular detection of infection with mycobacterium leprae

in Brazilian six banded armadillos (Euphractus sexcinctus). *Comparative Immunology, Microbiology and Infectious Diseases, 68*, 101397.
46. da Silva, M. B., Portela, J. M., Li, W., Jackson, M., Gonzalez-Juarrero, M., Hidalgo, A. S., et al. (2018). Evidence of zoonotic leprosy in Pará, Brazilian Amazon, and risks associated with human contact or consumption of armadillos. *PLoS Neglected Tropical Diseases, 12*(6), e0006532.
47. Urban, C., Blom, A. A., Pfrengle, S., Walker-Meikle, K., Stone, A. C., Inskip, S. A., et al. (2021). One health approaches to trace mycobacterium leprae's zoonotic potential through time. *Frontiers in Microbiology, 12*, 762263.
48. Lockwood, D., Butlin, C., & Penna, G. (2021). Current leprosy multi-drug treatment duration for MB patients (12 months) produces good clinical outcomes over many years. *Leprosy Review, 92*, 97–101.
49. World Health Organization. (2004). Twenty-five years of multidrug therapy for leprosy. *Weekly Epidemiological Record, 27*, 247–252.
50. Smith, C. S., Aerts, A., Saunderson, P., Kawuma, J., Kita, E., & Virmond, M. (2017). Multidrug therapy for leprosy: A game changer on the path to elimination. *The Lancet Infectious Diseases, 17*(9), e293–e2e7.
51. Dharmawan, Y., Fuady, A., Korfage, I., & Richardus, J. H. (2021). Individual and community factors determining delayed leprosy case detection: A systematic review. *PLoS Neglected Tropical Diseases, 15*(8), e0009651.
52. Dharmawan, Y., Fuady, A., Korfage, I. J., & Richardus, J. H. (2022). Delayed detection of leprosy cases: A systematic review of healthcare-related factors. *PLoS Neglected Tropical Diseases, 16*(9), e0010756.
53. Henry, M., GalAn, N., Teasdale, K., Prado, R., Amar, H., Rays, M. S., et al. (2016). Factors contributing to the delay in diagnosis and continued transmission of leprosy in Brazil--An explorative, quantitative, questionnaire based study. *PLoS Neglected Tropical Diseases, 10*(3), e0004542.
54. Schoenmakers, A., Mieras, L., Budiawan, T., & van Brakel, W. H. (2020). The state of affairs in post-exposure leprosy prevention: A descriptive meta-analysis on immuno- and chemo-prophylaxis. *Research and Reports in Tropical Medicine, 11*, 97–117.
55. Wang, H. (2024). Evidence of leprosy post exposure prophylaxis in highly endemic regions. *The Lancet Global Health, 12*(6), e905–e9e6.
56. Merle, C. S., Cunha, S. S., & Rodrigues, L. C. (2010). BCG vaccination and leprosy protection: Review of current evidence and status of BCG in leprosy control. *Expert Review of Vaccines, 9*(2), 209–222.

57. Wang, H. (2023). Leprosy vaccines: developments for prevention and treatment. In *Vaccines for neglected pathogens: Strategies, achievements and challenges [internet]* (pp. 47–69). Springer.
58. World Health Organization. (2015). Global leprosy update, 2014: Need for early case detection. *Weekly Epidemiological Record, 90*(36), 461–474.
59. World Health Organization. (2024). Global leprosy (Hansen disease) update, 2023: Elimination of leprosy disease is possible—Time to act! *Weekly Epidemiological Record, 37*, 501–510.
60. Anonymous. (2008). Global leprosy situation, beginning of 2008. *Weekly Epidemiological Record, 33*, 293–300.
61. World Health Organization. (2020). Global leprosy (Hansen disease) update, 2019: Time to step-up prevention initiatives. *Weekly Epidemiological Record, 95*, 417–438.
62. Smith, W. C., van Brakel, W., Gillis, T., Saunderson, P., & Richardus, J. H. (2015). The missing millions: A threat to the elimination of leprosy. *PLoS Neglected Tropical Diseases, 9*(4), e0003658.
63. Saunderson, P. R. (2008). Leprosy elimination: Not as straightforward as it seemed. *Public Health Reports, 123*(2), 213–216.
64. Kumar, M. S., Padmavathi, S., Shivakumar, M., Charles, U., Appalanaidu, M., Perumal, R., et al. (2015). Hidden leprosy cases in tribal population groups and how to reach them through a collaborative effort. *Leprosy Review, 86*(4), 328–334.
65. Vitiritti, B., Lima, F. R., de Castilho, N. T., Somensi, L. B., & Ogoshi, R. C. S. (2024). Hidden leprosy in a low-endemic area in southern Brazil: changes in endemicity following an active search. *The Brazilian Journal of Infectious Diseases, 28*(4), 103853.
66. Urgesa, K., Bobosha, K., Seyoum, B., Weldegebreal, F., Mihret, A., Howe, R., et al. (2021). Evidence for hidden leprosy in a high leprosy-endemic setting, eastern Ethiopia: The application of active case-finding and contact screening. *PLoS Neglected Tropical Diseases, 15*(9), e0009640.
67. Fernandes, T., Pereira, A. A., Cardoso, L. S., Alves Filho, V. P., Rezende Junior, L. S. N., & Souza, C. D. F. (2020). The hidden prevalence of leprosy: A comparative study between two Brazilian cities. *Revista da Associação Médica Brasileira, 66*(10), 1338–1343.
68. Mahato, R. K., Ghimire, U., Lamsal, M., Bajracharya, B., Poudel, M., Napit, P., et al. (2023). Evaluating active leprosy case identification methods in six districts of Nepal. *Infectious Diseases of Poverty, 12*(1), 111.

69. World Health Organization. (2021). *Towards zero leprosy: Global leprosy (Hansen's disease) strategy 2021–2030*. Regional Office for South-East Asia.
70. World Health Organization. (2019). Global leprosy update, 2018: Moving towards a leprosy free world. *Weekly Epidemiological Record, 35*(36), 389–412.
71. Henderson, D. A. (2011). The eradication of smallpox--an overview of the past, present, and future. *Vaccine, 29*(Suppl 4), D7–D9.
72. Cohen, J. (2023). Polio eradication effort struggles with end game. *Science, 381*(6664), 1271–1272.

Smallpox

Introduction

Smallpox was an ancient and much feared disease. It has been described as 'one of the greatest scourges of mankind'. The disease is highly infectious, causes a painful illness and has a high mortality rate. It is also non-discriminatory, killing kings and queens as well as the poor. The most distinctive feature of smallpox is the spots, blisters and pustules which first appear on the face and limbs and then cover the whole body. Smallpox derives its name from these spots (pox), with the adjective small being used to distinguish it from the great pox (syphilis) [1–3].

The most common form of smallpox, variola major, accounts for 90% of cases and has a case fatality rate of up to 30%. Most of those who survive are disfigured by pockmarks, extensive white scars, and many become blind. Variola minor is much less common, causes milder symptoms and has a fatality rate of 1%. There are two other rare forms of smallpox: the malignant and the haemorrhagic. These are almost always fatal. In the malignant form, patients have spots which remain soft and do not progress to become pustules. The haemorrhagic form initially presents as flat reddish areas that spread across the skin until they join up and darken. This form of the disease was often called the black pox or sledgehammer

© The Author(s), under exclusive license to Springer Nature Singapore Pte Ltd. 2025
I. K Crombie, *Major Pandemics*, https://doi.org/10.1007/978-981-95-2081-7_6

smallpox. It is caused extensive by bleeding into the skin and mucus membranes [4–6].

The Process of Infection

Smallpox is mainly spread by respiratory droplets from coughs, sneezes, although contact with clothing and bed linen contaminated with dried pustules can also lead to infection. There is also evidence that the disease can be transmitted over long distances in aerosols. In temperate climates smallpox outbreaks occur in the winter and early spring. A seasonal pattern is less obvious in tropical countries. In general, during cool and dry weather the frequency of infection increases [7, 8].

About 12 days after the initial exposure (range 7–17) patients have symptoms of headache, backache and a high fever. Then, as the patient is feeling better, a rash of flat red areas and small bumps appears, usually beginning on the face and then spreading across the body. After 1–2 days the bumps become filled with fluid. They then form crusty scabs which fall off after a few days [2, 4].

Origin and Spread

Smallpox is caused by a DNA virus named variola. It belongs to a group of pox viruses that includes horse-pox, cowpox, camelpox, taterapox (a disease of gerbils) and Mpox (formerly called monkeypox). Molecular genetic studies suggest that these viruses emerged sometime between 3000 and 6000 years. The variola virus that causes smallpox is probably younger and could have arisen between 1700 and 4000 years ago [9–11].

The region in which smallpox first emerged is unclear. It could have begun in Egypt or the Middle East, with humans acquiring the virus from camels or gerbils. A possible early case is the mummy of the Egyptian Pharaoh Rameses V who died just over 3000 years ago. He had pockmarks on his skin that resemble smallpox. Alternatively the disease may have originated in India or China [11–13].

Early Spread

If smallpox originated in Egypt, it could have spread along trade routes through Persia to India and then to China. Clinical descriptions of a disease that could be smallpox have been found in Sanskrit medical texts (the Charaka Samhita and Sushruta Samhita). These come from India and have been dated between 100 and 300 CE. Historical records suggest that smallpox may have spread to China around that time, reaching Japan and the Korean peninsula about 500 CE. Smallpox was likely to have been present in the Middle East in North Africa and Southern Europe at this time. The Arab invasions of Spain from 600 to 700 CE most likely increased the spread of smallpox. These early reports about smallpox and its spread need to be interpreted with caution. The first truly definitive description of the disease was not made until 910 CE by the Persian physician Abu Bakr al-Razi [9, 14, 15].

The Crusades, a series of religious wars between 1000 and 1300 CE, probably contributed to the spread of smallpox cases in Europe. The main aim of these wars was to reclaim Jerusalem and surrounding areas from the Muslims who lived there. After many battles, with wins and losses on both sides, the Christian troops finally withdrew permanently. At the end of each Crusade some of the returning troops could have carried smallpox to their home countries. As a result smallpox might have been transported across Europe [9, 14].

By 1500 CE reports of a disease that caused scarring on the face and body became increasingly common. In the 1600s smallpox started to feature in routinely collected data on causes of death in several European countries, and large outbreaks of smallpox were common. Even the rich and famous could be infected. In 1562 Queen Elizabeth I of England was left with facial scars and baldness that could have been caused by smallpox. Just over 100 years later, Queen Mary II of England died of smallpox [1, 14, 16].

Transported to the Americas

In the early 1500s slave ships from Africa carried smallpox to the Caribbean Islands. From there it quickly spread to Central America and to South America. Smallpox is often accused of contributing to the demise of the Aztec civilisation. In 1519, under the leadership of Hernán Cortés, the Spanish conquistadors invaded Mexico. The combination of troops armed with better weapons, such as crossbows, pistols and cannon, and an infectious disease (most likely smallpox) gifted the Spanish with an easy victory. However, historians disagree about the number of deaths smallpox caused and the consequences it had. Some claim that it killed millions of people, possibly up to 50% of the local population. Others seriously question the reliability these estimates, pointing out that in Europe in the 1500s smallpox was commonly regarded as a mild disease. The Aztecs were certainly conquered, and smallpox probably played a minor role [17, 18].

Smallpox was first introduced to Canada by French settlers in the 1500s. English and French fisherman probably took it to Martha's Vineyard, Massachusetts, in 1602. European settlers continued to bring the disease to the eastern seaboard of the United States. It spread rapidly among Native Indians, causing illness and death. There were also many outbreaks in towns on the East Coast, such as Boston, New York and Charleston in the mid-1600s. By the 1700s smallpox was well established across most of North America [19, 20].

The 1700s also witnessed another contentious event in the history of smallpox. The question is whether the British General Jeffery Amherst successfully launched a biological warfare attack on Native Indians in 1763. Letters sent between colleagues show that there was the intention to cause a large outbreak of smallpox by distributing blankets contaminated with dried pustules from smallpox victims. What is less clear is whether this act of biological warfare took place, and if it did, whether it was successful. The lack of 'ironclad evidence' on this issue has generated much speculation without producing a convincing answer [21].

Mortality Trends in Europe: 1600–1900

Official cause of death records for England, Finland and Sweden reveal a marked increase in smallpox mortality from 1600 to 1790. It is thought that a virulent new strain of the virus may have emerged in the mid-to-late 1600s. For example in London the proportion of deaths that were due to smallpox increased progressively from 2% in 1631 to 12% in 1721. Towns and cities across England recorded a similar high proportion of deaths from this disease in the mid-1770s. High mortality rates from smallpox were also reported in Sweden and Finland in the 1750s [22–24].

The remarkable rise in smallpox mortality was soon followed by an equally pronounced fall in death rates from about 1790 through to 1900. In London the proportion of deaths fell steeply to 3% in 1831, and by 1900 very few deaths were reported. Finland and Sweden experienced similar trends of death rates falling continuously from 1780 to low levels by 1900. These falls were not due to a reduction in disease severity. They were the result of the two interventions which provided immunity to infection, initially through the use of a technique known as variolation, and later by the introduction of the world's first vaccine [8, 22–24].

Preventing Smallpox

The first method for preventing smallpox was known in Europe as variolation. It was developed in China around 1000 CE, although acceptance of the technique was initially slow and it only became popular about 1500 CE. The process involved giving someone a mild disease to protect them against a more severe one. The Chinese described this as 'buying the flowers of heaven' with the flowers referring to the scars left by the mild disease. The method may have been based on careful observation: those with mild disease usually transmitted a mild infection to others. It could also have been influenced by the old idea that 'like cures like' or 'poison attacked by poison' [25, 26].

Variolation

The technique of variolation took crusty scabs from a person with mild disease, crushed them and then blew the powder into the patient's nostrils using a thin silver tube. Despite the initial reluctance to use this technique, the evident success in preventing severe smallpox gradually increased its popularity. Some treated patients did become ill and die, but the case fatality rate of 0.5–2% was substantially smaller than the 30% rate of natural infection. The technique spread from China and across Asia reaching Turkey in the seventeenth century and Europe in the early eighteenth century [27–29].

A key figure in bringing variolation to Britain was Lady Mary Worthley Montagu, the wife of the British Ambassador to Turkey. She was a noted society beauty whose looks had been scarred by smallpox. As a careful observer of Turkish customs and practices, she was impressed by the effectiveness of variolation. This led to her insisting that her five-year-old son receive the procedure in 1718. On returning to London, and against the strong advice of the College of Physicians, she had her daughter variolated as well. Her advocacy of the procedure encouraged the upper classes, and those of a scientific bent, to be variolated during the 1730s [27, 28, 30].

The use of variolation slowly increased in England until about 1750, after which its popularity boomed and mortality rates started to fall. Efforts were also made to ensure that the poor could also benefit from this preventive therapy. Then, just as it had become widely accepted, variolation was eclipsed by a more effective technique. This was developed by Edward Jenner, an English country doctor who had been variolated when he was 8 years old [27].

Vaccination

Jenner developed the first recognised human vaccine in 1796. As a country doctor, he was aware of the folktale that milkmaids were immune to smallpox. His own investigations confirmed that milkmaids who had contracted cowpox were protected against smallpox. To test this experimentally, Jenner took material from a pustule on the hand of Sarah Nelmes, a milkmaid with cowpox. He then transferred it to the arm of an eight-year-old boy, James Phipps, scratching the skin to allow the infection to penetrate. After a few weeks Jenner tried several times to induce a mild case smallpox using the technique of variolation, but the young Mr. Phipps was immune to the infection [31, 32].

Jenner's research was briefly halted because there was a shortage of milkmaids with cowpox. This forced him to take infective material directly from the pustules on cows' udders. (The term 'vaccination' comes from the Latin word *vacca*, meaning cow. It is now used for all types of vaccination, not just those derived from the udders of cows.) He also took material from horses because they suffered from a similar disease. Jenner conducted many further experiments on different people, using pustules from these animals as the main source of his vaccine. The viruses for cowpox, horse-pox and smallpox are all closely related, so vaccination with one of them provides immunity to the others [31, 32].

Jenner's early efforts were met with some criticism from his medical colleagues. Their views may have been influenced by the success of Jenner's method of vaccination, which threatened the livelihood of those doctors who used variolation. Some religious leaders also objected to vaccination, believing that it thwarted God's will by preventing disease. One well-publicised fear was that Jenner's use of fluid from pustules on cows would turn people into beasts. A famous cartoon by James Gilroy in 1802 portrayed patients who sprouted cows' heads from their faces, arms or buttocks. One unfortunate woman grew Satan-like horns on her head. Another picture from 1805 showed a boy with the face in the shape of the head of an ox. An organised campaign led by a Dr. Benjamin Moseley vociferously opposed vaccination. One of the claims was that this treatment would cause women to 'wander in the fields to receive the embraces of the bull' [3, 31–33].

Despite this opposition, the popularity of the vaccine grew rapidly, particularly after the publication of a report documenting the results from Jenner's study on 23 cases in 1798. In 1800, France, with the active encouragement of First Consul Napoleon Bonaparte, established a vaccine committee that investigated the safety and efficacy of Jenner's vaccine. Impressed by the results they made plans for a free national vaccination campaign. From France supplies of the vaccine were sent to Spain, where it quickly gained widespread support. The United States was also an early adopter of vaccination, with the then president, Thomas Jefferson, playing a leading role. Sweden began using the vaccine in 1801 and made it compulsory in 1816. Over that period the frequency of deaths from smallpox in Sweden fell from 2049 per million people to 133 per million. By 1890 the rate had fallen to 1 per million. In the early 1800s some German states enthusiastically adopted vaccination, with many making it compulsory. Others, like Prussia, used encouragement and the requirement that school pupils, apprentices and servants had to be vaccinated [3, 31, 34].

As well as vaccinating their own citizens, many European countries were concerned about the welfare of their overseas territories in the Americas and the Far East. The challenge here was to ensure that the vaccine material retained its potency during a long sea voyage. Vaccination was often conducted by collecting material from a pustule on an infected person and transferring it to another, the so-called arm-to-arm method. For sea voyages this was amended by the use of a group of orphan boys divided into pairs. One pair was vaccinated at the start of the voyage, followed by a new pair every 10 days until the destination was reached. Fortunately, other less ethically dubious techniques were also developed. These included drying the fluid from a pustule on a glass slide or using impregnated threads. Silver or ivory needles that had been coated fluid and dried were also popular. These techniques were not always effective, but they worked sufficiently often to enable local vaccination programmes to be conducted [27, 35].

To meet the growing demands for the vaccine, researchers Europe and the United States developed a method of large-scale production by using so-called vaccine farms. Young calves were inoculated several times, and material was collected when the pustules matured. This novel approached was welcomed because it overcame one of the hazards of direct arm-to-arm vaccination. That sometimes led to contamination by other disease such as syphilis and hepatitis [27, 31, 36].

Standardising the Vaccine

Until the twentieth century the vaccine industry comprised an unregulated mix of suppliers who derived their vaccines from undocumented sources. They could have obtained their material from any combination of cowpox, horse-pox, goat-pox and swinepox, as well as accidental contamination by human smallpox (variola virus). Added to this, the virus was often passed between animals (e.g. horse to cow) before being given to humans. Jenner thought that sequential transfer from horses to cows to humans produced the best vaccine. The material was also passed from human to animal to human. Surprisingly, and for reasons as yet unknown, a new virus emerged that was present in many of the vaccines in use in the early 1900s. This new virus was named vaccinia. Studies of samples of vaccines from the late 1800s showed that there were many different strains of vaccinia, and these were very closely related to the horse-pox virus [37–39].

The twentieth century brought in a new emphasis on standardisation of methods of vaccine production and strict quality control over all processes. The vaccinia virus was at the heart of this. In addition, the method of delivering the vaccine was also standardised. This led to steady improvements in the quality of the vaccine and to better techniques for vaccine storage. This was important for preserving the vaccine in tropical and semi-tropical countries where otherwise it would be inactivated by high temperatures. In one early technique, glycerol and lanolin were added to the fluid from pustules to increase the survival time of the stored vaccine. Another method was to scrape off the pustules from the skin of infected animals (cows or sheep) and dry the material under low pressure in the presence of sulphuric acid. But from the 1930s, freeze-drying of infective material provided a solution to long-term preservation of vaccine stocks. Adding peptone, a mixture of amino acids and fragments of proteins, to the vaccine fluid before freeze-drying preserved its potency even when used in tropical countries. These advances were a necessary prelude to the plans to eradicate smallpox from the world [37, 40].

When Smallpox Was Eradicated

With the availability of large quantities of low-cost, high-quality vaccines, serious thought was given to the global eradication of smallpox. The idea was not new. In 1801 Jenner predicted that smallpox, 'the most dreadful scourge of the human species', would be annihilated by the use of his vaccine. 5 years later Thomas Jefferson, president of the United States, wrote to congratulate Jenner on his discovery saying that 'Future nations will know by history only that the loathsome smallpox has existed and by you has been extirpated'. In the event it took another 177 years for eradication to be achieved [3, 41].

The argument for eradication was compelling. Smallpox was a major cause of serious illness and death. It was exclusively a human disease, so there was no animal reservoir which could restart epidemics. The vaccine was highly effective, easy to administer, and it conferred lifelong immunity. And the early mass vaccination campaigns had confirmed its effectiveness; by 1950 the infection had been eradicated from North America and most of Europe [42].

Global eradication was first proposed by the World Health Organization in 1953, but it was rejected as unrealistic. However the Pan American Sanitary Bureau decided to take the initiative, and some 5 years later had eliminated smallpox from all except four of the countries in South America. This may have prompted the USSR to table a new resolution on global eradication in 1959. It was approved by the World Health Assembly, but with such a small budget and so few staff that little progress was made. Then in 1966 WHO proposed an intensified eradication programme with an annual budget of $2.4 million which was to be supported by national budgets and voluntary donations. At that time smallpox cases were reported from 43 countries with more than 10 million cases and 2 million deaths each year. The intensified campaign began in 1967 and within 3 years smallpox had been eradicated in 20 West African countries. Key to this were the international donations of vaccine, particularly from the USSR and also the United States. By 1971 smallpox had been eradicated in South America. 2 years later the whole of Africa, except Ethiopia, was free of the disease [42–44].

Early in the campaign the aim had been to vaccinate between 80% and 100% of the population in countries with smallpox infections. Then experience in eastern Nigeria showed that the spread of the disease could be stopped by identifying outbreaks in their early stages and conducting mass vaccinations in each local area. This technique became known as ring vaccination in which everyone at risk of infection (i.e. within the ring) was to be treated. However, it relied on accurate reporting of cases, something that was poorly done. Resources were then diverted to appointing surveillance teams who urged local people to identify new smallpox outbreaks. Another innovation was the use of a forked needle to make a series of punctures in the skin. This method replaced other techniques because it was cheap, easy to use and very good at inducing immunity to smallpox [43].

There were setbacks. In 1972, four countries which had eliminated smallpox (Bangladesh, Botswana, Iran and Iraq) were reinfected by travellers from infected areas. By 1973 three of them were cleared of infection, although Bangladesh remained problematic. Outbreaks were also encountered in four other countries (Ethiopia, India, Nepal and Pakistan). This led to greatly intensified and well-resourced campaigns supported thousands of additional staff. Using techniques designed for densely populated areas, the Asian countries were cleared by 1975. This left Ethiopia, a vast and sparsely populated country with few roads and limited healthcare provision. A combination of volunteers and local staff transported by helicopter finally brought this pandemic to an end in 1976 [45].

Smallpox was finally officially extinguished from the world in 1978. The total cost of the programme was $298 million. High-income countries contributed $98 million, but then saved $350 million each year from 1978 because their populations no longer needed to be vaccinated. Low- and middle-income countries paid $200 million towards eradication. Their annual gains amounted to $1070 million because of the number of deaths that were avoided (about 1–2 million people died from smallpox each year). Clearly everyone gained from smallpox eradication, both financially and in lives saved. This was a landmark achievement and was rightly celebrated. It remains the only human disease ever to be eradicated [46].

Could Smallpox Return?

Smallpox may have been eradicated, but the threat of new outbreaks persists. Once the World Health Organization had confirmed that the virus had been extirpated eradicated, it recommended that all countries destroy their stocks of the virus. The aim was to prevent accidental leaks from research laboratories. Two leaks from laboratories in England, one in 1973 and the second in 1978, in which one person died, confirmed the risk. In 1977 some 18 laboratories were conducting research on smallpox, but by 1984 only two high-security facilities were designated to hold seedstocks of the virus: one in the United States and the other in Russia. These stocks could be used to generate vaccines in the event of a bioterrorist attack. But they also pose the risk of unintentional leaks of the virus. A gas explosion at the Russian facility in 2019 caused some structural damage, although no virus was released. The other concern is that there could be unofficial or even unintentional stockpiles of smallpox. Scientists found vials of smallpox virus that dated from 1950 in storage room of a laboratory in Maryland, United States, in July 2014. It is also suspected, but not known for certain, that several other countries may have maintained stocks of the virus [47–49].

The real concern is of a terrorist attack using smallpox as a biological weapon. This virus, along with anthrax, is judged to be the highest risk for bioterrorism. There are three frightening scenarios: smallpox could be sprayed into a building's air conditioning system, it could be spread in an airport concourse using a battery-powered hand-held nebuliser or a crop duster light aircraft could disperse it over crowds at a football game or a music festival. Once released the virus could spread quickly because everyone currently under the age of 50 is susceptible to the infection: they were all born after mass and local immunisation programmes had been terminated. Many of those aged over 50 may also be at risk as their level of immunity will have waned over time [50–52].

Licensed and unlicensed storage facilities are not the only potential source of the virus. Recent molecular genetic techniques have been used to create new versions of existing and ancient viruses from basic building blocks: all that is needed is the genetic code of the virus. To demonstrate the feasibility of this approach, Canadian researchers synthesised an extinct pox virus in 2017 using the basic building blocks of DNA. It would also be possible to manipulate the genetic code of the virus in what is called gain of function research. This could increase the virulence of the virus or make it immune to existing vaccines. The risk that researchers with malign intent could manufacture large quantities of 'improved' smallpox virus would seem small. It would require high levels of expertise and could take several years to achieve. The total cost would enormous, possibly billions of US dollars, well beyond the means of a few dissident scientists. However, such a strategy would not be beyond the means of a rogue nation. There is no evidence that unofficial stores of the virus exist or that renegade nation states are actively weaponising smallpox. But then no one is going to publicise such an abhorrent intention. Smallpox poses an ongoing threat, not so much 'gone but not forgotten', more the possibility of 'I'll be back' [48, 51, 53].

References

1. Behbehani, A. M. (1983). The smallpox story: Life and death of an old disease. *Microbiology Reviews, 47*(4), 455–509.
2. Kawalek, A., & Rudikoff, D. (2002). A spotlight on smallpox. *Clinics in Dermatology, 20*(4), 376–387.
3. Barquet, N., & Domingo, P. (1997). Smallpox: The triumph over the most terrible of the ministers of death. *Annals of Internal Medicine, 127*(8 Pt 1), 635–642.
4. Breman, J. G., & Henderson, D. A. (2002). Diagnosis and management of smallpox. *New England Journal of Medicine, 346*(17), 1300–1308.
5. World Health Organization. (2001). Smallpox: Forms of the disease. *Weekly Epidemiological Record, 76*, 337–344.
6. Soff, G. A., Levell, N. J., Parish, L. C., & Hoenig, L. J. (2023). British royalty and aristocracy: Their skin maladies part II. Queen Mary II'S death from hemorrhagic smallpox. *Clinics in Dermatology, 41*(6), 738–742.
7. MacIntyre, C. R., Das, A., Chen, X., Silva, C., & Doolan, C. (2019). Evidence of long-distance aerial convection of variola virus and implications for disease control. *Viruses, 12*(1), 33.
8. Krylova, O., & Earn, D. J. D. (2020). Patterns of smallpox mortality in London, England, over three centuries. *PLoS Biology, 18*(12), e3000506.
9. Thèves, C., Crubézy, E., & Biagini, P. (2016). History of smallpox and its spread in human populations. *Microbiology Spectrum, 4*, 4.
10. Babkin, I. V., Babkina, I. N., & Tikunova, N. V. (2022). An update of orthopoxvirus molecular evolution. *Viruses, 14*(2), 388.
11. Forni, D., Molteni, C., Cagliani, R., Clerici, M., & Sironi, M. (2023). Analysis of variola virus molecular evolution suggests an old origin of the

virus consistent with historical records. *Microbial Genomics, 9*(1), mgen000932.
12. Li, Y., Carroll, D. S., Gardner, S. N., Walsh, M. C., Vitalis, E. A., & Damon, I. K. (2007). On the origin of smallpox: Correlating variola phylogenics with historical smallpox records. *Proceedings of the National Academy of Sciences of the United States of America, 104*(40), 15787–15792.
13. Berche, P. (2022). Life and death of smallpox. *La Presse Médicale, 51*(3), 104117.
14. Fenner, F., Henderson, B., Arita, I., et al. (1988). *The history of smallpox and its spread around the world. Smallpox and its eradication* (pp. 209–244). World Health Organisation.
15. Brüssow, H. (2023). Pandemic potential of poxviruses: From an ancient killer causing smallpox to the surge of monkeypox. *Microbial Biotechnology, 16*(9), 1723–1735.
16. Carmichael, A. G., & Silverstein, A. M. (1987). Smallpox in Europe before the seventeenth century: Virulent killer or benign disease? *Journal of the History of Medicine and Allied Sciences, 42*(2), 147–168.
17. Alden, D., & Miller, J. C. (1987). Out of Africa: The slave trade and the transmission of smallpox to Brazil, 1560-1831. *Journal of Interdisciplinary History, 18*(2), 195–224.
18. Brooks, F. (1993). Revising the conquest of Mexico: Smallpox, sources, and populations. *Journal of Interdisciplinary History, 24*, 1–29.
19. Bianchine, P. J., & Russo, T. A. (1992). The role of epidemic infectious diseases in the discovery of America. *Allergy and Asthma Proceedings, 13*(5), 225–232.
20. Beach, W. (1885). Contagions and epidemics in America. *JAMA, 4*, 281–285.
21. Fenn, E. A. (2000). Biological warfare in eighteenth-century North America: Beyond Jeffery Amherst. *Journal of American History, 86*(4), 1552–1580.
22. Mercer, A. (1985). Smallpox and epidemiological-demographic change in Europe: The role of vaccination. *Population Studies, 39*, 287–307.
23. Sköld, P. (1996). From inoculation to vaccination: Smallpox in Sweden in the eighteenth and nineteenth centuries. *Population Studies, 50*(2), 247–262.
24. Pitkänen, K. J., Mielke, J. H., & Jorde, L. B. (1989). Smallpox and its eradication in Finland: Implications for disease control. *Population Studies, 43*(1), 95–111.

25. Summers, W. C. (1994). Congruences in Chinese and Western medicine from 1830-1911: Smallpox, plague and cholera. *Yale Journal of Biology and Medicine, 67*(1–2), 23–32.
26. Cai, J. (1998). A historical overview of traditional Chinese medicine and ancient Chinese medical ethics. *Ethik in der Medizin, 10*, S84–S91.
27. Fenner, F., Henderson, D., Arita, I., et al. (1988). Early efforts at control: Variolation, vaccination, and isolation and quarantine. In *Smallpox and its eradication [internet]* (pp. 245–276). World Health Organization. https://iris.who.int/handle/10665/39485
28. Dinc, G., & Ulman, Y. I. (2007). The introduction of variolation 'a La Turca' to the west by Lady Mary Montagu and Turkey's contribution to this. *Vaccine, 25*(21), 4261–4265.
29. Jacobs, B. L., Langland, J. O., Kibler, K. V., Denzler, K. L., White, S. D., Holechek, S. A., et al. (2009). Vaccinia virus vaccines: Past, present and future. *Antiviral Research, 84*(1), 1–13.
30. Grundy, I. (2000). Montagu's variolation. *Endeavour, 24*, 4–7.
31. Henderson, D. A. (1997). Edward Jenner's vaccine. *Public Health Reports, 112*(2), 116–121.
32. Esparza, J., Nitsche, A., & Damaso, C. R. (2018). Beyond the myths: Novel findings for old paradigms in the history of the smallpox vaccine. *PLoS Pathogens, 14*(7), e1007082.
33. Lee, D., & Fulford, T. (2000). The beast within: The imperial legacy of vaccination in history and literature. *Literature and History, 9*(1), 1–23.
34. Edwardes, E. J. (1902). A century of vaccination: Small-pox epidemics and small-pox mortality before and since vaccination came into use. *British Medical Journal, 2*(2166), 27–30.
35. Mark, C., & Rigau-Pérez, J. G. (2009). The world's first immunization campaign: The Spanish smallpox vaccine expedition, 1803-1813. *Bulletin of the History of Medicine, 83*(1), 63–94.
36. Esparza, J., Lederman, S., Nitsche, A., & Damaso, C. R. (2020). Early smallpox vaccine manufacturing in the United States: Introduction of the "animal vaccine" in 1870, establishment of "vaccine farms", and the beginnings of the vaccine industry. *Vaccine, 38*(30), 4773–4779.
37. Fenner, F., Henderson, D., Arita, I., et al. (1988). Developments in vaccination control between 1900 and 1966. Smallpox and its eradication. In *History of international public health* (pp. 277–314). World Health Organization.

38. Souza, A. R. V., Brinkmann, A., Esparza, J., Nitsche, A., & Damaso, C. R. (2023). Gene duplication, gene loss, and recombination events with variola virus shaped the complex evolutionary path of historical American horsepox-based smallpox vaccines. *MBio, 14*(5), e0188723.
39. Qin, L., Favis, N., Famulski, J., & Evans, D. H. (2015). Evolution of and evolutionary relationships between extant vaccinia virus strains. *Journal of Virology, 89*(3), 1809–1824.
40. Collier, L. H. (1955). The development of a stable smallpox vaccine. *Journal of Hygiene, 53*(1), 76–101.
41. Geddes, A. M. (2006). The history of smallpox. *Clinics in Dermatology, 24*(3), 152–157.
42. Fenner, F. (1982). A successful eradication campaign. Global eradication of smallpox. *Reviews of Infectious Diseases, 4*(5), 916–930.
43. Henderson, D. A. (1975). Smallpox eradication—the final battle. *Journal of Clinical Pathology, 28*(11), 843–849.
44. Henderson, D. A. (2011). The eradication of smallpox—an overview of the past, present, and future. *Vaccine, 29*(Suppl 4), D7–D9.
45. Henderson, D. A. (1987). Principles and lessons from the smallpox eradication programme. *Bulletin of the World Health Organization, 65*(4), 535–546.
46. Barrett, S. (2013). Economic considerations for the eradication endgame. *Philosophical Transactions of the Royal Society, B: Biological Sciences, 368*(1623), 20120149.
47. Williams, R. E. (1981). In pursuit of safety. *Journal of Clinical Pathology, 34*(3), 232–239.
48. MacIntyre, C. R. (2020). Reevaluating the risk of smallpox reemergence. *Military Medicine, 185*(7–8), e952–e9e7.
49. McCarthy, M. (2014). Smallpox samples are found in FDA storage room in Maryland. *BMJ, 349*, g4545.
50. Green, M. S., LeDuc, J., Cohen, D., & Franz, D. R. (2019). Confronting the threat of bioterrorism: Realities, challenges, and defensive strategies. *The Lancet Infectious Diseases, 19*(1), e2–e13.
51. Jane, J. (2009). Smallpox as a weapon for bioterrorism. In K. A. Fong (Ed.), *Bioterrorism and infectious agents: A new dilemma for the 21st century* (pp. 147–167). Springer.
52. Heymann, D. L. (2004). Smallpox containment updated: Considerations for the 21st century. *International Journal of Infectious Diseases, 8*(Suppl 2), S15–S20.

53. Shinomiya, N., Minari, J., Yoshizawa, G., Dando, M., & Shang, L. (2022). Reconsidering the need for gain-of-function research on enhanced potential pandemic pathogens in the post-COVID-19 era. *Frontiers in Bioengineering and Biotechnology, 10*, 966586.

Cholera: The Recurring Pandemic

Introduction

Over the past 200 years, cholera has caused seven major pandemics that have wreaked destruction around the world. The last one to do so began in earnest in 1961 and is still active today. In 2023 about 535,000 cholera cases and 4000 deaths were reported to the World Health Organization (WHO). As only 5–10% of cases are reported to WHO, the true number of cases will be very much greater [1–3].

The bacterium, *Vibrio cholerae*, is responsible for cholera. It can cause acute diarrhoea. Fortunately, about 80% of people who are infected with *V. cholerae* do not have any symptoms. Those who do become ill usually have a mild form of the disease that resolves in a few days. But about one in five of symptomatic cases has severe disease. These unfortunates suffer from profuse, foul diarrhoea and vomiting, accompanied by agonising abdominal cramps. Within a few hours healthy individuals can become weak, sunken-eyed and then comatose. Some die within 12 hours after symptoms begin and others linger for a few days. Severe disease results from a profuse emission of watery diarrhoea, often described as rice-water stools (colourless fluid with flecks of mucous). This causes a loss of fluid, up to 1 L/h, leading to severe dehydration, very low blood pressure, acute

© The Author(s), under exclusive license to Springer Nature Singapore Pte Ltd. 2025

I. K Crombie, *Major Pandemics*, https://doi.org/10.1007/978-981-95-2081-7_7

renal failure, breathlessness and loss of consciousness. Without treatment about 50% of those with severe dehydration die [4].

In the nineteenth century cholera was commonly called it *la mort de chien* (the dog's death) because of the unpleasantness of dying. The term 'cholera' is most likely derived from two Greek words meaning flow and bile; an ancient theory (the doctrine of humours) held that an excess of bile could cause disease. However, the term could also come from the Greek word for a gutter, likening the main symptom of the disease to the rush of water in gutters during rainstorms [5–7].

Why it Causes Disease

V. cholerae is an accidental killer. Normally the bacterium lives a quiet, unassuming life in river deltas, such as the Bay of Bengal, absorbing nutrients and multiplying. It particularly likes attaching to the shells of crustaceans (crabs, shrimps, prawns and particularly tiny copepods) because it digests chitin, the main constituent of the shells. To be able to cause disease *V. cholerae* has to acquire several genes that transform it into a virulent bacterium. Two of these genes are particularly important. One of them contains the information for the cholera toxin which is responsible for the severe diarrhoea suffered by cholera victims. The DNA for the cholera toxin comes from bacteriophage (a virus that attacks bacteria) known as CTXΦ. The other, toxin coregulated pilus (TCP), is essential for the survival and the multiplication of the bacterium in the small intestine [8, 9].

In the Bay of Bengal, the process of becoming a virulent bacterium probably begins with heavy rainfall that carries nutrients from the land into rivers and out into the shallow seas. An abundance of nutrients causes a bloom of phytoplankton, which provide a food source for the tiny copepods. These tiny animals also multiply rapidly, creating a plentiful supply of chitin for *V. cholerae*. This stimulates a rapid increase in the number of bacteria. The bacteriophage CTXΦ also multiplies because there are lots of *V. cholerae* to infect. This increases the chances that it will donate the toxin gene to the bacterium. *V. cholerae* can also accept new bits of DNA from its neighbours through a process called horizontal gene transfer. An abundance of chitin primes the bacteria to receive the new DNA. Several transfer events provide the bacterium with the other genes needed for toxicity, making it ready to cause pandemics [9–11].

Beliefs About the Cause

Religions around the world were united in the view was that cholera was a punishment for sinful behaviour that offended the god(s), although the reasoning involved and the responses of the faithful varied. Hindus in India thought that the actions of the British colonisers transgressed their beliefs and angered their gods. Buddhists believed that demigods had been angered and that wearing protective amulets and pilgrimages to shrines would protect against disease. Sunni Muslims considered cholera outbreaks as a test of faith and adopted a fatalistic approach to the disease. Shi'ite Muslims saw cholera as a punishment for sin that could be ameliorated by praying for deliverance and wearing talismans inscribed with holy verses. Christians of all denominations saw cholera as divine punishment for sin, with prayers and penitence as the only protection. Some Christian groups identified the specific sins, such as indolence, gambling and drunkenness, and suggested that these indulgences weakened the body, predisposing it to disease. In England, cholera was thought to be a visitation of Divine Providence, attacking those who were addicted to spirits or indulged in 'irregular and sensual habits'. The United States had a similar view, although was more specific, welcoming the high death rate among female sex workers as an appropriate punishment for their sins. It is ironic that religion, at least the mass gatherings for religious festivals, contributed to the high mortality in India and in Moslem countries [12–14].

The Six Nineteenth-Century Pandemics

Cholera has a long and close association with the Indian subcontinent. The Sushrata Samita, a Sanskrit text from 500 BCE, describes a disease that closely resembles cholera. Alexander the Great may have encountered cholera when his army invaded north-western India in 327 BCE. Vasco da Gama, the Portuguese explorer who discovered the sea route to India, was also aware of a disease that was probably cholera. One of his officers, Gaspar Correa, described an outbreak of acute gastro-intestinal disease in 1503 which killed 20,000 people, some of them dying within 8 hours of the symptoms appearing. A further 64 outbreaks of cholera in the Indian subcontinent were reported by Europeans between 1503 and 1817. None of these had spread far beyond the Indian subcontinent. But cholera was about to change. The year 1816 had been unusually hot and dry while 1817 experienced very heavy rainfall and disastrous floods. This was when a virulent new form of the disease rampaged across India and well beyond its borders [1, 7, 15].

The First Pandemic 1817–1823

The first pandemic began in Jessore on the river Ganges in 1817. It quickly spread across India killing up to 2 million people, making it one of the most terrible of cholera epidemics. This vigorous new disease travelled along overland trade routes and sea routes: east to Myanmar, Thailand, China, Japan and the Philippines, and west to the Middle East, Turkey and Egypt. Soldiers returning home from two wars, the Oman conflict and the battles between Persia and Turkey, accelerated the spread of cholera. The westward journey of the pandemic stalled at Astrakhan in southeast Russia, just to the north of the Caspian Sea. Further progress was probably prevented by the very severe winter of 1823/24. But the rapid spread of the disease and the humiliating and agonising process of dying raised concern in the European countries which had substantial trade with Asia [6, 13, 15, 16].

The Second Pandemic: 1826–1851

European countries did not have to wait long for their concerns to be realised: the second pandemic began in Bengal in 1826. It followed the same routes as the first pandemic, eastward to China and westward to

Afghanistan in 1828/29, reaching Persia and south-east Russia by the late summer of 1829. After a pause over the winter of 1829, the disease travelled from Russia to the Baltic countries. Its spread was aided by the Russian troops who invaded Poland in response to an uprising in 1830. Another source of spread was among pilgrims to Mecca in 1831. Many took cholera with them as they returned to their home countries of Syria, Palestine, Egypt and Tunisia [15].

From the Baltic countries cholera spread across mainland Europe, through Austria to Germany 1931, arriving in Belgium and France in 1832 and Spain in 1833. It was carried to England in 1831 from the German and Baltic ports, particularly Hamburg and Riga. In 1832 cholera was transported by ship to North America, along the St Lawrence Seaway, first to Quebec then onto New York and Philadelphia. It spread across the United States. eventually reaching the Pacific coast in 1833. In the same year Spanish sailors took the disease to Cuba, and by 1837 it had invaded Central America. After its dramatic spread around much of the world, this pandemic settled into a routine of causing sporadic outbreaks in countries previously visited as well as invading several new ones. The outbreaks in England and Wales in 1848–1849 killed over 50,000 people, making it the worst they had experienced [6, 15, 17, 18].

The second pandemic cholera also generated social discontent and conspiracy theories. At its core was the belief that the high death rate among the poor was the result of a plot by those in power to cull those less fortunate. In many countries people believed that the poor were being poisoned by doctors who were well paid for their work. The resulting cholera riots were widespread, from New York to Russia. They were also frequent; for example, there were 72 riots in Britain between 1831 and 1833. A variation on the conspiracy theory in British cities was that doctors were killing patients to supply bodies for medical studies. This idea probably came from the well-publicised trial of Burke and Hare, two murderers in Edinburgh who were convicted in 1828 for supplying bodies for medical dissection [17, 19].

The Third to Sixth Pandemics

The next four pandemics also originated in the Bengal region and largely followed the same routes as the second pandemic. However, they generated few riots. Possibly a new, mysterious and deadly disease can promote social unrest and violence. But when that illness reappears after a brief absence, familiarity may make it tolerable. The exceptions to this were Russia and to a lesser extent Italy. They stand out as having cholera riots until the end of the nineteenth century with violence targeted towards government officials and the police as well as doctors. The brutal suppression of the uprisings in these two countries probably sustained the resentment of the poor, driving them to riot [17, 19, 20].

The third pandemic (1852–1859) devastated countries in the Middle East and was particularly severe in Russia, where over one million people died. Southern Europe escaped serious harm, although countries in the north fared less well. Japan was also badly hit with about 200,000 deaths in an outbreak in Tokyo that began in 1858 [15, 18, 20].

The main feature of the fourth pandemic (1863–1879) was that more countries were affected than in any other pandemic. Italy suffered particularly badly with over 150,000 deaths. A pilgrimage to Mecca led to 30,000 cases of cholera and subsequently to many deaths in Turkey, the Middle East and Russia when the pilgrims returned to their home countries [13, 15, 17, 20, 21].

The fifth pandemic (1881–1896) was largely a mild affair with limited impact on Western Europe, North Africa and the Americas. Pilgrims returning from Mecca may have been responsible for a large outbreak in Egypt in 1883, which may have caused 58,000 deaths. Cholera was particularly severe in Russia, with about 800,000 people dying of it between 1892 and 1894 [13, 15, 17, 20, 21].

The sixth pandemic (1899–1923) had very little impact on Western Europe, although Italy, and particularly Naples, suffered outbreaks. Emigrants from Italy to the United States may have carried the disease across the Atlantic. The worst outbreaks were in Asia, particularly India, although Russia was also badly affected with over 200,000 deaths. Small outbreaks of this sixth pandemic continued to occur sporadically, and the movement of troops in the First World War helped spread the disease [13, 15, 17, 20, 21].

Contagion, Quarantine and Miasma

In the early nineteenth century, cholera was thought to be contagious because it travelled along overland trade routes and shipping routes. It was also spread by invading armies and organised pilgrimages. The belief that travellers spread the disease led the European countries to impose quarantines at the onset of the second pandemic. Since the Black Death, quarantine had been the standard method for preventing the spread of deadly diseases. Ships that came from places where cholera was present could be refused entry to ports and overland travellers from such regions were supposed to be isolated in special buildings (lazarettos) [22].

Although many European countries implemented systems of quarantine, only a few countries, such as Spain and Britain, attempted to enforce these regulations. In consequence, quarantine failed to prevent the spread of the disease, and it was abandoned. At this time eminent medical authorities thought that cholera was not contagious. For example, in 1849 the Royal College of Physicians, London, and the Board of Health in Dublin issued statements that carers in the home and doctors in hospital were not at risk of contracting the disease [22–24].

Many other causes of cholera were proposed in the first half of the nineteenth century. The telluric theory held that a poison exuded from the earth was responsible. Others suggested that atmospheric electricity or a shortage of ozone were the cause. But by far the most popular was the zymotic theory. It took different forms. One proposed that some chemicals in the air became unstable due to the action of heat, electricity or friction, and underwent a form of fermentation. This created a miasma, corrupted air, that caused disease. A variation on this theme was that the miasma was generated by rotting animal and vegetable matter. This version became the dominant for most of the nineteenth century [25–27].

Cholera and Miasma in Britain

Evidence that appeared to confirm miasma as the cause of cholera came from a landmark study in the 1830s into the living conditions of the working people in Britain. It showed that cholera mortality was highest in localities with uncleared heaps of rubbish and cesspits that overflowed with stagnant urine and faeces. As drainage systems were poor or non-existent, liquid oozed from this waste seeping into ditches, canals and streams. These conditions were thought to generate the miasma that led to cholera. They also explained why the poor suffered such a high mortality from cholera [28, 29].

London, then the most densely populated city in the world, faced a crisis of waste disposal in the mid-1800s. Cesspits, and the noxious odours that they produced, attracted most of blame for the severe cholera outbreak in 1848–1849. Drastic action was needed, and the response was to ban all cesspools in London. Over a six-year period, some 30,000 cesspits were replaced by a system of sewers which fed into the rivers that flowed beneath London. These were natural rivers that had been built over as the city expanded. They all fed into the River Thames. This solved the problem of cesspits and was supposed to get rid of the disease-causing miasma. But it also transported the faeces of people with cholera into the Thames. Unfortunately, this river was the main source of London's drinking water [30–32].

The most important consequence of the new sewer system was the Great Stink of 1858. That year the summer had been hot and dry and a foul stench powerful enough to bring tears to the eyes hung over London. The Thames is a tidal river and at low tide human excreta were deposited on the mud banks where they rotted in the sun. The smell was so offensive that the Houses of Parliament were closed to protect the health of MPs from the supposedly deadly effects of this miasma. Politicians, the press and the public were outraged by this foul corrupting air. In response, the government allocated £3.5 million, then a colossal sum, to create a comprehensive sewerage system for London. Under the direction of Joseph Bazalgette, 450 miles of main sewers, and 13,000 miles of smaller local sewers were built between 1859 and 1865. This transported human excreta and other waste matter 14 miles downstream of central London. More than 150 years later that system is still in use today [30–32].

London was not unique in having a great stink; Paris had two. A foul stench that pervaded the city in 1880 created outrage among Parisians. Because of the dominance of the miasma theory, the smell was labelled 'a potentially dangerous health hazard'. Three factors caused the stink: defective cesspits, the illegal dumping of cesspit contents into sewers and problems with the treatments plants that processed human excrement. Attempts were made to install proper sewage systems, but these were vigorously opposed by some national and municipal officials, the press and the *vidangeurs* (those who cleaned the cesspits). As a result, the offensive smells afflicted Paris again in 1895. However, this time its citizens were merely offended, the fear of deadly diseases was no longer present; the true cause of cholera had been identified a few years earlier [33, 34].

Identifying the Cause

The miasma theory remained dominant for most of the 1800s, although a few far-sighted doctors thought otherwise. John Snow was a London-based doctor who based his ideas on clinical observations. He conducted several studies during the second and third pandemics that convinced him and some colleagues that cholera was not caused by foul-smelling miasma. Among other findings he showed that water taken from a heavily polluted part of the Thames was eight times more likely to lead to death from a cholera than cleaner water taken from further upstream [26].

Snow's findings were interesting, but they failed to convince most doctors and politicians. When the fourth pandemic struck London in 1866, the majority view was that miasma was to blame, with overcrowding and immoral sensual habits increasing susceptibility to the disease. Variation in mortality rates between different sources of water was attributed to differences in the soil from which the water was extracted. This theory was proposed by one Max von Pettenkoffer. He was a highly influential and virulent critic of Snow's suggestion of a poison spread by water [35, 36].

Identification of the true cause of cholera had to await the general acceptance of the germ theory of disease. Louis Pasteur was the genius who showed that microscopic organisms caused illness in chickens, pigs and sheep as well as humans. But it was the acclaimed German scientist Robert Koch who finally established in 1884 that *Vibrio cholerae* was responsible for cholera. He showed that *V. cholerae* could be identified in all the patients who had the disease and that it was present in sufficient numbers to explain all the symptoms. He was also able to grow the bacterium in culture media. The miasma theory was finally defeated and Koch was awarded the Nobel Prize. But the last word should go to Max von Pettenkoffer, a champion of environmental health and hygiene and a dedicated anticontagionist. In 1892, at the age of 74, he drank a fresh culture of *Vibrio cholerae* and suffered only a mild diarrhoea. To him it was proof that the bacterium alone did not cause the disease; it had to be modified by passing through the right kind of soil. Nowadays we would think he was one of the lucky ones who only had a mild illness [37–39].

How it Is Spread

Cholera is a disease spread by poor hygiene and inadequate sanitary facilities. People acquire the infection by consuming water or foodstuffs contaminated with *V. cholerae*. On being swallowed the acid conditions in the stomach kill off most of the bacteria. A large number of *V. cholerae*, about 100 million, need to be ingested for some survivors to make it through to the small intestine where they can multiply rapidly. The conditions in the stomach determine whether enough bacteria will make it through to the intestines. A high level of stomach acidity reduces the chances of survival, whereas poor diet and malnutrition increase it. Further, some foodstuffs, such as rice, fish, custard and skimmed milk, neutralise the stomach acid so that even low doses of bacteria can thrive [40–42].

During the infection, the bacterium is expelled with the faeces. The rice-water stools that characterise severe disease contain about 100 million *V. cholerae* per ml (millilitre). On average, those with cholera excrete the bacterium for about 2 days, but some people do so for up to 14 days.

When these bacteria come into contact raw fruit and vegetables or with cooked food, they multiply rapidly. Raw seafood and undercooked shellfish also feature frequently as a source of infection. Within a few hours foodstuffs can attain large enough numbers of *V. cholerae* to ensure that the infection spreads [40, 42–44].

The Seventh Pandemic

The seventh pandemic began in the Middle East. A new strain of *V. cholerae* was first identified in 1905 at a quarantine station in the village of El Tor in Egypt. It was isolated from Indonesian pilgrims returning from Mecca. As was the custom at the time, the strain was named after the village where it was found. Early in its career, the El Tor strain was infectious but did not cause severe disease. Its ancestor had come from Bengal at some time in the past, and the new strain probably emerged in the Middle East about 1897 [45, 46].

The sequence of events by which El Tor achieved virulence is quite different from that of the first six pandemics. It had picked up a few extra genes in Egypt by 1908. Then in the 1920s it travelled to Sulawesi, one of the larger islands of Indonesia. Here it gained the rest of the genes and mutations needed to make it highly infectious and moderately virulent. Four small outbreaks in Sulawesi between 1937 and 1958 heralded the onset this latest pandemic. But it only began in earnest in 1961, spreading first to neighbouring Indonesian islands and then on to Bengal. From this ancestral home of cholera, El Tor rampaged round the world in three overlapping waves, infecting millions of people [45–47].

It travelled around Southeast Asia before making its way westwards through India, Pakistan and Russia, reaching the Middle East and Africa in 1970. The following year it invaded Europe where it caused some small outbreaks, with the largest affecting about 2000 people. El Tor then made a dramatic entry into S. America in 1991. From an initial outbreak in Peru, the infection spread to almost every country in Central and South America, causing over one million cases and 12,000 deaths [47–49].

Africa, particularly sub-Saharan Africa, stands out as the region most blighted by the seventh pandemic. Cholera arrived in West Africa in 1970. Initially only 11 countries were affected but it quickly spread across sub-Saharan Africa and by the early 2000s Africa had 94% of global cases. Although case number gradually reduced, a global map of cholera cases between 2008 and 2012 confirmed the predominance of cholera in African countries [2, 6, 50].

Natural and Man-Made Disasters

Many of the major outbreaks of cholera in the seventh pandemic were driven by extreme climate events. Heavy rainfall can cause flooding that washes out open-air defecation sites and overwhelms sewage systems. This leads to contamination of sources of drinking water and the unwitting consumption of the cholera bacterium. India, Bangladesh and many countries in sub-Saharan Africa are at risk of this type of outbreak [51–53].

Paradoxically cholera outbreaks in India, Bangladesh and sub-Saharan Africa often follow severe droughts. Zimbabwe suffered such outbreaks in 2008 and 2018. Water shortages can lead to poor handwashing and lower standards of personal hygiene. Lack of water to flush toilets means people have to defecate in the bush, allowing cholera to seep into local rivers. In addition, severe drought may cause people to migrate to other regions. In 1991–1992 an estimated 1.3 million people were forced to move from Mozambique to Zimbabwe. There they were housed in overcrowded refugee camps with limited sanitation facilities leading to large outbreaks of cholera [51–53].

Another natural disaster, a devastating earthquake, hit Haiti in January 2010, displacing over 1 million people and destroying essential infrastructure such as water supplies and sewage disposal. But it was the arrival of United Nations peacekeepers from Nepal that caused Haiti's first cholera outbreak in 100 years. They brought the cholera bacterium with them. By 2019, over 800,000 people developed cholera and at least 10,000 people died, with many deaths unrecorded. In recognition of the central role of the UN peacekeepers, the Secretary General of the United

Nations formally begged the Haitian people for forgiveness in 2016 [54, 55].

Armed conflict also exacerbates cholera outbreaks. In 1994 about one million people fleeing from genocide in Rwanda were housed in overcrowded conditions in Zaire (now the Democratic Republic of Congo). Limited supplies of clean water and poor sewage disposal caused a cholera outbreak in which at least 50,000 became ill. Another large outbreak struck Nigeria in 2021. The effects of flooding and a shortage of clean water were exacerbated by armed conflict involving Boko Haram and criminal gangs. Millions of people were displaced into overcrowded facilities, making a major outbreak of cholera was inevitable. Over 100,000 people developed cholera and 3600 died [52, 56–58].

One of the largest cholera outbreaks in recent history was due to the combination of risk factors. For many years Yemen has been one of the world's poorest countries. It suffered from lack of clean drinking water, poor sanitation and malnutrition. Then a civil war in 2014 destroyed much of the country's infrastructure, particularly the healthcare facilities. A cholera outbreak between 2016 and 2019 caused 2 million cases and 4000 deaths [59, 60].

Environmental Reservoirs

The Ganges river delta was the ultimate source, the environmental reservoir, from which the nineteenth-century cholera pandemics sprang. But the global spread of cholera during the seventh pandemic may have created other aquatic reservoirs. Genetic studies in Haiti after the 2010 catastrophe suggest that the El Tor strain may have established reservoirs which can seed new outbreaks. Aquatic reservoirs have been suggested as the source of many the recent outbreaks in Africa. Most cases of the disease occurred in landlocked countries far from the sea, with infections being particularly common around the Great African Lakes and the Lake Chad Basin. If reservoirs are sources of new outbreaks, substantial investment in clean drinking water and efficient sewage systems would be needed to prevent repeated epidemics of cholera [52, 61, 62].

Medical Advances to Reduce Mortality

Two medical advances have greatly reduced the impact of cholera outbreaks, oral rehydration therapy and a vaccine. Effective oral rehydration therapy to replace the fluid and the salts lost through severe diarrhoea was gradually developed in the twentieth century. A method suitable for use in field settings became available for worldwide use in the late 1970s. Swift use of this therapy can reduce the mortality rate in severe cholera from over 50% to less than 1%. It has saved countless thousands of lives. Most remarkably oral rehydration therapy is very effective in reducing mortality in the group most at risk, children under 5 years. It is often combined with antibiotics, particularly for patients with severe disease. Several antibiotics are available for use, although only as an adjunct to rehydration therapy. Their effectiveness is gradually being eroded as the bacterium develops antibiotic resistance [63, 64].

Research to develop a cholera vaccine began in the 1860s, but it was not until 1991 that an oral vaccine was licensed for use. It has the advantage of inducing an immune response on the surface of the intestines, the place where *V. cholerae* multiplies. The vaccine is administered in two doses and provides protection to 50–80% of immunised adults. The level of protection falls substantially within 3–5 years. Children under 5 years gain less benefit from the vaccine. The vaccines have to be kept cold, 2–8 ° C, so can only be used in settings which can provide refrigeration. Several other types of vaccine are being developed in an effort to overcome these limitations [65–67].

When Will It End?

Devastating pandemics of cholera that travel around the world in waves of infection are almost certainly a thing of the past. Although it is always possible that a new highly infectious and virulent strain will appear, the physical environment in which the bacterium used to thrive has largely disappeared. During the course of the nineteenth and twentieth centuries, clean water supply and sewage disposal systems were gradually installed in Europe, the Americas, most of Asia and much of Africa. All the high-income and most of the middle-income countries now provide the water and sewage disposal systems that prevent the disease from spreading [68].

What is likely to continue for the foreseeable future are repeated large outbreaks in many low-income countries. Environmental reservoirs that seed new outbreaks, together with poverty and its many consequences, are the main causes. The contributing factors are: [61, 69–71].

- Shortage of clean drinking water, lack of facilities for handwashing and poor sanitation disposal spread cholera infection. Population growth and increased urbanisation exacerbate these problems.
- Insufficient healthcare premises, shortage of trained staff and limited supplies of vaccines and rehydration fluids impede prevention and treatment.
- Reluctance to seek healthcare, in part due to poor literacy and to distrust of national and local authorities, reduces access to treatment and vaccination.
- Inadequate capacity for surveillance and outbreak detection allows small outbreaks to grow.
- Climate change and extreme weather events can spread infection. Flooding can contaminate drinking water; drought can force reliance on dirty water and prevent proper handwashing.
- Earthquakes and wars can destroy sanitation systems, force mass population movement to makeshift camps with inadequate water and sanitation facilities

In response to these challenges a Global Task Force on Cholera Control was launched in 2017. At that time about 2.9 million cases and 95,000 deaths occurred each year. The strategy focused on the 47 countries that suffer from repeated cholera outbreaks, with the aim of reducing deaths by 90% and eliminating the infection in 20 countries by 2030. The strategy has three pillars [72, 73]:

- detect outbreaks early using the recently developed rapid diagnostic tests.

- tackle cholera hotspots through targeted mass vaccination campaigns and by improving supplies of clean water and sewage disposal systems.
- provide the resources and technical support to ensure that local communities have the capacity and skills to identify outbreaks quickly and implement appropriate control measures.

Delivering these aims will be challenging. The first shipment of 1.2 million rapid diagnostic tests was only delivered, to Malawi, in April 2024. The vaccine supply falls far of what is needed. For example in 2022 it was estimated that 74 million doses were needed but only 35 million were available. It is hoped the annum level of production will increase to 50 million in 2024. However, the Task Force target of 1.5 billion doses to be delivered by 2030 is unlikely to be met. Another problem is that there have been decades of underinvestment in the provision of water supply and sewage disposal. The result is that 2 billion people lack access to clean drinking water and 3.6 billion do not have safely managed sanitation. Finally, it is not clear who will provide the resources and technical support needed for training local staff [74–77].

Although some progress has been made towards the Task Force goals, it is clearly not enough. In 2023 the World Health Organization issued an urgent call for substantial new investment in cholera control. This was in response to 'an unprecedented surge of cholera outbreaks across the world'. Thirty countries experienced this increase in cases, and an estimated one billion people are at moderate to high risk of contracting the disease. At present the global infrastructure for preventing and controlling cholera infection appears inadequate. More importantly, until measures are put in place to tackle poverty and poor sanitation, large cholera outbreaks are destined to continue [78–80].

References

1. Siddique, A. K., & Cash, R. (2014). Cholera outbreaks in the classical biotype era. *Current Topics in Microbiology and Immunology, 379*, 1–16.

2. Ali, M., Nelson, A. R., Lopez, A. L., & Sack, D. A. (2015). Updated global burden of cholera in endemic countries. *PLoS Neglected Tropical Diseases, 9*(6), e0003832.
3. World Health Organisation. (2024). Cholera, 2023. *Weekly Epidemiological Record, 36*, 481–495.
4. Davies, H. G., Bowman, C., & Luby, S. P. (2017). Cholera - management and prevention. *The Journal of Infection, 74*(Suppl 1), S66–s73.
5. Howard-Jones, N. (1974). Cholera nomenclature and nosology: A historical note. *Bulletin of the World Health Organization, 51*(3), 317–324.
6. Lacey, S. W. (1995). Cholera: Calamitous past, ominous future. *Clinical Infectious Diseases, 20*(5), 1409–1419.
7. Colwell, R. R. (1996). Global climate and infectious disease: The cholera paradigm. *Science, 274*(5295), 2025–2031.
8. Childers, B. M., & Klose, K. E. (2007). Regulation of virulence in vibrio cholerae: The ToxR regulon. *Future Microbiology, 2*(3), 335–344.
9. Kumar, A., Das, B., & Kumar, N. (2020). Vibrio pathogenicity Island-1: The master determinant of cholera pathogenesis. *Frontiers in Cellular and Infection Microbiology, 10*, 561296.
10. Jutla, A. S., Akanda, A. S., Griffiths, J. K., Colwell, R., & Islam, S. (2011). Warming oceans, phytoplankton, and river discharge: Implications for cholera outbreaks. *The American Journal of Tropical Medicine and Hygiene, 85*(2), 303–308.
11. Islam, M. S., Islam, M. S., Mahmud, Z. H., Cairncross, S., Clemens, J. D., & Collins, A. E. (2015). Role of phytoplankton in maintaining endemicity and seasonality of cholera in Bangladesh. *Transactions of the Royal Society of Tropical Medicine and Hygiene, 109*(9), 572–578.
12. Phillips, H. (2020). '17, '18, '19: religion and science in three pandemics, 1817, 1918, and 2019. *Journal of Global History, 15*, 434–443.
13. Stewart-Tull, D. E. (2001). Vaba, Haiza, Kholera, Foklune or cholera: In any language still the disease of seven pandemics. *Journal of Applied Microbiology, 91*(4), 580–591.
14. Briggs, A. (1961). Cholera and society in the nineteenth century. *Past & Present, 19*, 76–96.
15. Pollitzer, R. (1954). Cholera studies. 1. History of the disease. *Bulletin of the World Health Organization, 10*(3), 421–461.
16. McGrew, R. (1960). The first cholera epidemic and social history. *Bulletin of the History of Medicine, 34*, 61–73.

17. Evans, R. J. (1988). Epidemics and revolutions: Cholera in nineteenth-century Europe. *Past Present, 120*, 123–146.
18. Ramamurthy, T., & Ghosh, A. (2021). A re-look at cholera pandemics from early times to now in the current era of epidemiology. *Journal of Disaster Research, 16*, 110–117.
19. Cohn, S. K. (2017). Cholera revolts: A class struggle we may not like. *Social History, 42*(2), 162–180.
20. Patterson, K. D. (1994). Cholera diffusion in Russia, 1823-1923. *Social Science & Medicine, 38*(9), 1171–1191.
21. Arnold, D. (1986). Cholera and colonialism in British India. *Past & Present, 113*, 118–151.
22. Tognotti, E. (2013). Lessons from the history of quarantine, from plague to influenza a. *Emerging Infectious Diseases, 19*(2), 254–259.
23. Altemira, D. (1885). Cholera and quarantine. *Lancet, 124*, 88–89.
24. Graves, R. J. (1849). On the progress of asiatic cholera. *Dublin Quarterly Journal of Medical Science, 7*(13), 1–39.
25. Halliday, S. (2002). Commentary: Dr john Sutherland, vibrio cholerae and 'predisposing causes'. *International Journal of Epidemiology, 31*(5), 912–914.
26. Snow, S. J. (2002). Commentary: Sutherland, snow and water: The transmission of cholera in the nineteenth century. *International Journal of Epidemiology, 31*(5), 908–911.
27. Ackerknecht, E. H. (2009). Anticontagionism between 1821 and 1867: The fielding H. Garrison lecture. 1948. *International Journal of Epidemiology, 38*(1), 7–21.
28. Lilienfeld, D. E. (1978). "the greening of epidemiology": Sanitary physicians and the London epidemiological society (1830-1870). *Bulletin of the History of Medicine, 52*(4), 503–528.
29. Fee, E., & Brown, T. M. (2005). The public health act of 1848. *Bulletin of the World Health Organization, 83*(11), 866–867.
30. Davenport, R. J., Satchell, M., & Shaw-Taylor, L. M. W. (2019). Cholera as a 'sanitary test' of British cities, 1831-1866. *The History of the Family, 24*(2), 404–438.
31. Tynan, N. (2013). Nineteenth century London water supply: Processes of innovation and improvement. *The Review of Austrian Economics, 26*, 73–91.
32. Cook, G. C. (2001). Construction of London's Victorian sewers: The vital role of Joseph Bazalgette. *Postgraduate Medical Journal, 77*(914), 802–804.
33. Barnes, D. S. (2002). Scents and sensibilities: Disgust and the meanings of odors in the late nineteenth-century Paris. *Historical Reflections, 28*(1), 21–49.

34. Soppelsa, P. (2009). Finding fragility in Paris: The politics of infrastructure after Haussmann. *Journal of the Western Society for French History, 37*, 233–247.
35. Luckin, W. (1977). The final catastrophe--cholera in London, 1866. *Medical History, 21*(1), 32–42.
36. Lippi, D., & Gotuzzo, E. (2014). The greatest steps towards the discovery of vibrio cholerae. *Clinical Microbiology and Infection, 20*(3), 191–195.
37. Bordenave, G. (2003). Louis Pasteur (1822-1895). *Microbes and Infection, 5*(6), 553–560.
38. Gillies, D. A. (2016). Establishing causality in medicine and Koch's postulates. *International journal of history and philosophy of medicine, 6*, 1–13.
39. Evans, A. S. (1973). Pettenkofer revisited: The life and contributions of max von Pettenkofer (1818-1901). *The Yale Journal of Biology and Medicine, 46*(3), 161–176.
40. Nelson, E. J., Harris, J. B., Morris, J. G., Jr., Calderwood, S. B., & Camilli, A. (2009). Cholera transmission: The host, pathogen and bacteriophage dynamic. *Nature Reviews. Microbiology, 7*(10), 693–702.
41. Cash, R. A., Music, S. I., Libonati, J. P., Snyder, M. J., Wenzel, R. P., & Hornick, R. B. (1974). Response of man to infection with vibrio cholerae. I. Clinical, serologic, and bacteriologic responses to a known inoculum. *The Journal of Infectious Diseases, 129*(1), 45–52.
42. Estrada-García, T., & Mintz, E. D. (1996). Cholera: foodborne transmission and its prevention. *European Journal of Epidemiology, 12*(5), 461–469.
43. Taylor, D. L., Kahawita, T. M., Cairncross, S., & Ensink, J. H. (2015). The impact of water, sanitation and hygiene interventions to control cholera: A systematic review. *PLoS One, 10*(8), e0135676.
44. Richterman, A., Sainvilien, D. R., Eberly, L., & Ivers, L. C. (2018). Individual and household risk factors for symptomatic cholera infection: A systematic review and meta-analysis. *The Journal of Infectious Diseases, 218*(suppl_3), S154–s164.
45. Cvjetanovic, B., & Barua, D. (1972). The seventh pandemic of cholera. *Nature, 239*(5368), 137–138.
46. Hu, D., Liu, B., Feng, L., Ding, P., Guo, X., Wang, M., et al. (2016). Origins of the current seventh cholera pandemic. *Proceedings of the National Academy of Sciences of the United States of America, 113*(48), E7730–e7739.
47. Mutreja, A., Kim, D. W., Thomson, N. R., Connor, T. R., Lee, J. H., Kariuki, S., et al. (2011). Evidence for several waves of global transmission in the seventh cholera pandemic. *Nature, 477*(7365), 462–465.

48. Oprea, M., Njamkepo, E., Cristea, D., Zhukova, A., Clark, C. G., Kravetz, A. N., et al. (2020). The seventh pandemic of cholera in Europe revisited by microbial genomics. *Nature Communications, 11*(1), 5347.
49. Domman, D., Quilici, M. L., Dorman, M. J., Njamkepo, E., Mutreja, A., Mather, A. E., et al. (2017). Integrated view of vibrio cholerae in the Americas. *Science, 358*(6364), 789–793.
50. Gaffga, N. H., Tauxe, R. V., & Mintz, E. D. (2007). Cholera: A new homeland in Africa? *The American Journal of Tropical Medicine and Hygiene, 77*(4), 705–713.
51. Rieckmann, A., Tamason, C. C., Gurley, E. S., Rod, N. H., & Jensen, P. K. M. (2018). Exploring droughts and floods and their association with cholera outbreaks in sub-saharan Africa: A register-based ecological study from 1990 to 2010. *The American Journal of Tropical Medicine and Hygiene, 98*(5), 1269–1274.
52. Rebaudet, S., Sudre, B., Faucher, B., & Piarroux, R. (2013). Environmental determinants of cholera outbreaks in inland Africa: A systematic review of main transmission foci and propagation routes. *The Journal of Infectious Diseases, 208*(Suppl 1), S46–S54.
53. Charnley, G. E. C., Kelman, I., & Murray, K. A. (2022). Drought-related cholera outbreaks in Africa and the implications for climate change: A narrative review. *Pathogens and Global Health, 116*(1), 3–12.
54. Piarroux, R., Moore, S., & Rebaudet, S. (2022). Cholera in Haiti. *Presse Médicale, 51*(3), 104136.
55. Hadeed, S. J., Broadway, K. M., Schwartz-Watjen, K. T., Tigabu, B., Woodards, A. J., Swiatecka, A. L., et al. (2022). Notional spread of cholera in Haiti following a natural disaster: Considerations for military and disaster relief personnel. *Military Medicine, 188*, e2074–e2081.
56. Shackleton, D., Memon, F. A., Nichols, G., Phalkey, R., & Chen, A. S. (2023). Mechanisms of cholera transmission via environment in India and Bangladesh: State of the science review. *Reviews on Environmental Health, 39*, 313–329.
57. Gulumbe, B. H., Yusuf, Z. M., Faggo, A. A., et al. (2023). The interplay among conflict, water scarcity, and cholera in northern Nigeria. *Public Health Challenges, 2*, e118.
58. Elimian, K., Yennan, S., Musah, A., Cheshi, I. D., King, C., Dunkwu, L., et al. (2022). Epidemiology, diagnostics and factors associated with mortality during a cholera epidemic in Nigeria, October 2020-October 2021: A

retrospective analysis of national surveillance data. *BMJ Open, 12*(9), e063703.
59. Tarnas, M. C., Al-Dheeb, N., Zaman, M. H., & Parker, D. M. (2023). Association between air raids and reported incidence of cholera in Yemen, 2016-19: An ecological modelling study. *The Lancet Global Health, 11*(12), e1955–e1963.
60. Simpson, R. B., Babool, S., Tarnas, M. C., Kaminski, P. M., Hartwick, M. A., & Naumova, E. N. (2022). Dynamic mapping of cholera outbreak during the Yemeni civil war, 2016-2019. *Journal of Public Health Policy, 43*(2), 185–202.
61. Islam, M. S., Zaman, M. H., Islam, M. S., Ahmed, N., & Clemens, J. D. (2020). Environmental reservoirs of vibrio cholerae. *Vaccine, 38*(Suppl 1), A52–a62.
62. Mavian, C. N., Tagliamonte, M. S., Alam, M. T., Sakib, S. N., Cash, M. N., Moir, M., et al. (2023). Ancestral origin and dissemination dynamics of reemerging toxigenic vibrio cholerae, Haiti. *Emerging Infectious Diseases, 29*(10), 2072–2082.
63. Guerrant, R. L., Carneiro-Filho, B. A., & Dillingham, R. A. (2003). Cholera, diarrhea, and oral rehydration therapy: Triumph and indictment. *Clinical Infectious Diseases, 37*(3), 398–405.
64. Hassoun, S., Leasu, F., Manu, P., Rogozea, L. M., Dinu, E., & Cocuz, M. E. (2023). Pharmacological management of cholera: A century of expert opinions in Cecil textbook of medicine. *American Journal of Therapeutics, 30*(6), e519–e525.
65. Sit, B., Fakoya, B., & Waldor, M. K. (2022). Emerging concepts in cholera vaccine design. *Annual Review of Microbiology, 76*, 681–702.
66. Deen, J., Holmgren, J., & Clemens, J. D. (2022). Evaluating improved inactivated oral cholera vaccines for use in ending endemic cholera by 2030: Opportunities and challenges. *The Lancet Infectious Diseases, 22*(10), e292–e298.
67. World Health Organization. (2017). Cholera vaccines: WHO position paper—August 2017. *Weekly Epidemiological Record, 92*(34), 477–498.
68. Abellan, J. (2017). Water supply and sanitation services in modern Europe:developments in 19th-20th centuries. In *XII international congress of the Spanish association of economic history*. Universidad De Salamanca.
69. Ajayi, A., & Smith, S. I. (2019). Recurrent cholera epidemics in Africa: Which way forward? A literature review. *Infection, 47*(3), 341–349.

70. D'Mello-Guyett, L., Gallandat, K., Van den Bergh, R., Taylor, D., Bulit, G., Legros, D., et al. (2020). Prevention and control of cholera with household and community water, sanitation and hygiene (WASH) interventions: A scoping review of current international guidelines. *PLoS One, 15*(1), e0226549.
71. Amisu, B. O., Okesanya, O. J., Adigun, O. A., Manirambona, E., Ukoaka, B. M., Lawal, O. A., et al. (2024). Cholera resurgence in Africa: Assessing progress, challenges, and public health response towards the 2030 global elimination target. *Le Infezioni in Medicina, 32*(2), 148–156.
72. Legros, D. (2018). Global cholera epidemiology: Opportunities to reduce the burden of cholera by 2030. *The Journal of Infectious Diseases, 218*(suppl_3), S137–s140.
73. Global Task Force on Cholera Control. (2017). *Ending cholera: A global roadmap to 2030.* http://www.who.int/cholera/publications/global-roadmap.pdf?ua=1
74. Feinmann, J. (2023). Cholera makes a comeback amid calls to boost vaccine production. *BMJ, 380*, 636.
75. Memish, Z. A., Blumberg, L., Al-Maani, A. S., Baru, R., Dube, E., Gao, G. F., et al. (2024). Moving cholera vaccines ahead of the epidemic curve. *Lancet, 403*(10422), 127–129.
76. UN-Water. (2023). *The United Nations world water development report 2023: Partnerships and cooperation for water.* United Nations.
77. Jesudason, T. (2024). Global action to improve access to tools for cholera. *The Lancet Infectious Diseases, 24*(6), e361.
78. World Health Organisation. (2023). *Call for urgent and collective action to fight cholera.* World Health Organisation.
79. Olu, O. O., Usman, A., Ameda, I. M., et al. (2023). The chronic cholera situation in Africa: Why are African countries unable to tame the well-known lion? *Health Services Insights, 16*, 11786329231211964.
80. Panda, S., Chatterjee, P., Deb, A., Kanungo, S., & Dutta, S. (2020). Preventing cholera in India: Synthesizing evidences through a systematic review for policy discussion on the use of oral cholera vaccine. *Vaccine, 38*(Suppl 1), A148–A156.

Polio

Introduction

For most of human history, polio was a rare disease. It was called infantile paralysis because it mainly attacked very young children, causing lifelong severe weakness of the muscles in the legs or the arms. The Scottish poet and novelist, Sir Walter Scott, was most likely one of those rare cases. In 1773, at 18 months of age, he had a fever that lasted 3 days and resulted in paralysis of one leg. Polio also has a more sinister side. In a small proportion of cases, the muscles that control breathing are so seriously impaired that the patient dies [1, 2].

The origins of polio are obscure. Sporadic pieces of evidence suggest rather than confirm its presence. The oldest is the skeleton of an Egyptian mummy from 3700 BCE who had a shortening of the left leg suggestive of polio. More convincing is a stone carving from ancient Egypt (about 1500 BCE). It shows a priest with a shortened and withered leg, and a foot which hangs loosely, classic signs of paralytic polio. An ancient Greek vase from about 500 BCE depicts a man with a withered left leg and a spinal deformity, possibly a consequence of paralytic polio. Many centuries later, a sketch of a beggar by Heironymous Bosch (1450–1516) also portrays the withering of a leg that could indicate polio [2–4].

© The Author(s), under exclusive license to Springer Nature Singapore Pte Ltd. 2025

I. K Crombie, *Major Pandemics*, https://doi.org/10.1007/978-981-95-2081-7_8

Detailed clinical descriptions of polio do not appear until late in the eighteenth century. In 1789, the paediatrician Michael Underwood described many of the features of polio. He recognised that it mainly affected young children. The disease began with a fever that led to severe weakness mainly in the lower limbs, particularly the left leg. Then in 1840 the German orthopaedist Jakob Klein published data on a series of 27 cases and defined the clinical features of polio. He also showed that paralytic polio was probably caused by damage to the spinal cord. Although polio mainly affected young children, it was not considered an important disease at that time [2, 4, 5].

The Early Polio Outbreaks

Views on polio had changed across the nineteenth century because clusters of cases began to appear. The isolated island of St Helena and the town of Worksop in England were the first to experience small groups of cases in 1836. In the following decades several other clusters of cases were reported. Norway experienced its first outbreak in 1868, involving 14 cases, 12 of whom were children. Subsequently northern Sweden had an outbreak of 18 cases in 1881, followed by a larger one with 43 cases in Stockholm in 1887. Then in 1899 the Norwegian town of Bratsburgh reported 54 cases, with a similar number occurring in the same year in Stockholm. Starting in 1893, the United States experienced small outbreaks almost every year, punctuated with moderate ones, such as the 132 cases in Vermont in 1894. Other industrialised countries—Germany, Austria, Holland, Switzerland, England and Australia—also reported small outbreaks in the late 1800s [2, 5–7].

Levels of concern grew as the size of the outbreaks increased in the early years of the twentieth century. Over the 2 years 1905–1906 both Norway and Sweden experienced over 1000 cases, and Germany reported over 1000 cases in 1909. In the United States there were 2500 cases in New York in 1907, and 923 in Massachusetts in 1909. By the early 1900s most of Europe and the United States and Canada, had reported large outbreaks of polio. The largest recorded outbreak began in New York in 1916 and spread across the northeast corner of the United States. Of the

20,000 cases, almost 9000 occurred in New York. In panic, parents moved an estimated 50,000 children out of the city to less dangerous places [7–9].

In subsequent decades, countries across Europe experienced large outbreaks every 5–10 years. In the United States more moderate outbreaks occurred on an annual basis until 1944 when the number of cases increased each year, rising to a peak of 55,825 cases across the whole country in 1952. A feature of these outbreaks is that they occurred in late summer to early autumn, the same time as apples ripened on trees. In Sweden this led to the fear that windfalls of that fruit caused polio and to the health warning: 'Do not eat those apples; they've been on the ground'. The industrialised countries were in the grip of a new pandemic [5, 6, 10, 11].

In low–and middle-income countries the picture was quite different. Paralytic polio was rare in places as India and China in the early part of the twentieth century. In Puerto Rico, El Salvador and Mauritius, medium-sized outbreaks did not appear until the 1930s. Even in the 1950s, few countries in Africa had more than 100 cases over a 5-year period. None of these countries experienced outbreaks approaching the scale of those seen in Europe and North America [12, 13].

Finding the Cause

For most of the nineteenth century infantile paralysis was thought to be due to teething, foul bowels or a fever. Another view, proposed by Sir William Osler in his celebrated 1892 *Textbook of Medicine*, was that paralytic polio was caused by a minor injury. Although small outbreaks occurred, the general view for much of the nineteenth century was that polio did not behave like an infectious disease. If it were, then it should spread most readily in close family members; but in most family groups only one person succumbed to the illness. Then, towards the end of the nineteenth century, research studies began to suggest that polio could be infectious. With hindsight it is obvious that teething and minor injuries could not explain the sudden emergence of outbreaks that gradually increased in size [11, 14, 15].

A careful investigation by Ivor Wickman and colleagues confirmed that polio was infectious. They studied an outbreak of over 1000 cases in Sweden in 1905 that were spread across several villages. This showed that polio only spread to a new village if it had been visited by someone from an infected village. Further if two villages were separated by a physical barrier, such ravine or unpassable river, the disease was never transmitted from one to the other. Finally in one village, Traestena, most of the cases of polio were in children who had attended the local school. This suggested that polio was infectious. But a surprising finding was that many of those exposed to polio did not develop symptoms of disease. Studies in the United States a few years later replicated the findings of the Swedish study. It also clarified that a high proportion of those infected with polio show no symptoms. This is the reason for the apparent lack of transmission within families in the Swedish study. Most of them were infected, but few developed symptoms of the disease [14, 16, 17].

The final, slightly gruesome, step in identifying the cause of polio was made in Vienna in 1908. Two scientists, Landsteiner and Popper, took extracts from the spinal cord of polio victims. They passed the fluid through a filter that would trap bacteria, then injected it into the brains of two monkeys. Both developed polio. As only a virus could pass through the filter, then a virus must be the cause of the disease. This experiment confirmed that polio was infectious [18].

How Polio Spreads

Following the discovery that polio was caused by a virus, an American research group led by Simon Flexner investigated how polio entered the body. In 1910 they showed that when samples of the virus were rubbed on the nasal passage on monkeys, the animals subsequently developed polio. Their conclusion was that the virus entered nerves in the nose and then migrated to the spinal cord. So strongly did this group propose that the virus began replicating in nerve cells in the nose that other experimental evidence was ignored for the next 20 years. This included the findings of a Swedish group: in 1912 Kling and colleagues isolated the virus from the small intestine. Although it suggested that the nose was not the only region in which the virus replicated, this possibility was not pursued. It was not until the early 1930s that other American groups confirmed that the virus initially grew in the cells lining the oesophagus and the intestines and subsequently spread to nerve cells. They also showed that the virus was present in human faeces and in sewage. The conclusion was that the polio virus enters via the mouth, multiplies in the digestive system and is excreted in faeces. This meant that the infection can be spread by consuming food or water contaminated by faeces. It can also be contracted by swimming in contaminated water [17, 19].

The Biology of Infection

Infection begins when the virus invades and replicates in the cells lining the back of the throat and then migrates to the intestines where it continues to multiply. The virus is then excreted in the faeces of infected individuals, usually for 3–4 weeks, although sometimes it may continue for 5–6 weeks. Most cases occur by consuming objects contaminated with faeces. The virus can also be spread by respiratory secretions, but this is much less common [20–22].

Most of those infected will experience no symptoms, and only about 25% develop flu-like symptoms (headache, sore throat and fever). Up to 5% will experience neck stiffness and pain in the back and legs. These symptoms last for just over a week. In about 1% of those infected, the virus invades cells in the spinal cord, destroying the nerves that control the muscles and causing paralysis in the arms or legs. Usually only one limb is affected [21, 22].

Only a tiny minority of patients have an infection which damages the nerves that control breathing. Untreated most of these individuals die unless they are given some form of mechanical ventilation. The first such machine was the iron lung. The patient was placed inside a large cylinder with pumps which repeatedly compressed the lungs, allowing breathing to occur. The machine was large, unpleasant for the patient, and very few were available for use. A major improvement in the form of positive pressure ventilation device was introduced by a team of Danish doctors in 1952. It reduced the mortality rate from 87% to 26% and was soon manufactured in sufficient quantities to meet patient needs. More sophisticated machines which are smaller and more user-friendly have since been developed [23, 24].

Explaining Apparent Changes in the Behaviour of the Virus

The trend from isolated cases to small, then large and finally very large outbreaks among industrialised countries suggested that something about polio infection was changing. This trend began in the mid-nineteenth century and accelerated in the twentieth century. It followed a geographical sequence from Scandinavia to many other countries in Northern Europe and then to North America. Another notable feature of polio was the change in the age of the cases. Prior to 1890 the disease occurred predominantly among infants and young children, with 90% of cases in those under 5 years. Starting in the twentieth century the age at onset gradually increased, and this change followed the same geographical pattern as the large outbreaks. Further, the switch to increasing age also happened more quickly in urban areas and among those of higher socioeconomic status [14, 25–27].

The apparent change in the behaviour of the virus had an unexpected cause. It was most likely due to the trend among industrialised countries to install high-quality sanitation facilities in houses and apartments. Improvements in hygiene usually reduce the frequency of infectious diseases, but the reverse may be true for polio. The explanation is straightforward. Babies up to 6 months of age were protected from infection by maternal antibodies transferred in breast milk. This protective effect gradually waned as the infants aged, so that everyone over the age of 6 months was at risk of contracting polio. With the basic sanitation facilities in the late nineteenth century most people would be infected while they were still young and would experience no symptoms or very mild ones. These children would have lifelong protection against polio. But with higher standards of sanitation, older children and some adults would not have acquired an immunity to polio when very young. They would be at risk of contracting polio as they mixed with their peers, leading to large outbreaks and an increasing age at infection. This explanation is also consistent with the absence of large outbreaks of polio in low–and middle-income countries during the mid-nineteenth to mid-twentieth centuries. As Paul commented, 'those countries which pride themselves on having advanced standards of sanitation and low infant mortality rates have the highest poliomyelitis rates' [13, 14, 28, 29].

The Impact of the Vaccine

Among high-income countries the frequency of polio cases plummeted dramatically in the 1960s and continued to fall in the 1970s. This was the result of using effective vaccines in mass immunisation programmes. As there are three strains of the virus, imaginatively labelled types I, II and III, vaccines had to be able to provide immunity to all of them. The first vaccine was developed by Jonas Salk in the late 1940s. It contained a mix of all three types of poliovirus which had been inactivated (killed) by treatment with formalin. A very large randomised controlled trial involving over half a million children showed the vaccine to be effective. The findings were reported on 12 April 1955: it gave 68% protection against type I polio, 100% against type II and 92% against type III. Because supplies had been stockpiled in anticipation of a positive result, vaccine distribution began in the United States on 13 April 1955. A few weeks later vaccination distribution was stopped. Vaccines from one manufacturer, Cutter Laboratories, had caused polio among at least 200 of those vaccinated. Further research showed that this was due to inadequate inactivation of the virus. In response the manufacturing process was amended to ensure this accident could not be repeated. The inactivated polio virus (IPV) was safe for use in countries across the world [30, 31].

But the inactivated polio virus (IPV) had weaknesses. It had to be administered by injection on four occasions, and it had only a moderate impact on the type I virus, the most common cause of infection. Independently of Salk, the Polish American scientist Albert Bruce Sabin developed a different type of vaccine. His early research had shown that the virus entered the body through the mouth and replicated in the intestinal tract. Sabin developed a vaccine that mimicked the natural course of infection. First the virus was severely weakened (attenuated) so that it would not cause disease. Then the vaccine was administered by mouth so that it could replicate in the intestines. Tests with monkeys and chimpanzees showed that it provided high levels of protection against all three types of polio virus. Permission to conduct a formal clinical trial in the United States was denied because the mass immunisation campaign meant there was a shortage of vaccine naive subjects. There were also concerns that there might be a repeat of the Cutter debacle. Instead, it was tested in Northern Ireland, the Congo and the Soviet Union [32–34].

This attenuated vaccine included all three types of virus, and proved to be highly effective against polio. Because it was administered by mouth, initially in a sugar cube, it was called oral polio vaccine (OPV). This vaccine acted more quickly and produced longer-lasting immunity than the inactivated Salk vaccine. By multiplying in the intestines, the attenuated virus created an immunological barrier that greatly reduced viral transmission by the faecal/oral route. The advantages of higher effectiveness, low production costs and easier administration led the United States to switch to the oral vaccine in 1961. The World Health Organization also recommended the new vaccine, and most countries in the world began using it. Although Sabin was encouraged to patent his vaccine and become very rich, he declined. Preferring to keep the price low so that everyone could benefit, he explained: 'It's my gift to the world's children' [31–34].

Experience in the Americas

In the United States mass immunisation against polio began in the early 1950s, initially with Salk's inactivated vaccine and then from 1961 with Sabin's attenuated one. The effect was dramatic. Within 20 years the annual number of cases fell from just over 10,000 to just over 10. Cuba had similar success with its nationwide vaccination campaign, reducing the case numbers from just less than 400 per year in 1959 to zero in 1962. Then in 1975 Brazil adopted a program of national immunisation days that reduced the number of cases from 2330 to 122 in 1981. These successes encouraged the countries of the Americas to adopt a goal of eliminating the infection across the whole region. Although initially there were mixed views on the wisdom of this approach, the plan was accepted. By 1991 mass vaccination campaigns had eliminated polio from the region [35–38].

The Global Eradication Campaign

Inspired by the success of smallpox eradication campaign, and the impressive progress made in controlling polio in the Americas, the World Health Organization launched the Global Polio Eradication Campaign in 1988. This was a far greater challenge than that faced by the Americas, so a longer time was allowed: the aim was to free the world from polio by the year 2000. The campaign had four strategies. To conduct mass immunisation campaigns to achieve 90% coverage in all countries. To hold national immunisation days vaccinating all children under 5 years. To monitor for outbreaks of polio and vaccinate all children under 5 years in the affected area. And finally to conduct mopping up vaccinations in areas where new cases among young children had emerged in the previous 3 years [39].

The combined effect of the four strategies was to reduce the number of polio infections from 350,000 in 1988 to 3500 in 2000. This was a tremendous achievement, and, although eradication had not been achieved, there was hope that it was imminent. This appeared justified. By 2002, the Americas, Western Pacific and European Regions were certified polio-free, and by 2005 only four countries—India, Nigeria, Pakistan and Afghanistan—had polio cases caused by the original (wild type) virus. The polio eradication campaign was entering the endgame [40, 41].

The Endgame

The experience from the successful eradication of smallpox was that mopping up the last few cases was difficult. For the polio the task is proving even more challenging. One problem is that the oral vaccine was less effective in many low- and middle-income countries. For some reason the three types of polio virus in the vaccine appeared to interact, reducing overall effectiveness. This was exacerbated by failure to vaccinate, particularly in areas of high population density. Armed conflicts in several regions also impeded the work of immunisation teams, leaving many thousands of children without protection against infection. For example the Yemen, which was polio-free between 2009 and 2015, suffered polio outbreaks between 2019 and 2022. This was a result of conflict between the Houthi regime in the north and the government in the south. Vaccination teams were unable to access some areas, and in some districts in the north vaccination was banned by the local authorities [41–43].

Vaccine refusal was a serious issue in some countries. Misplaced beliefs about the harms of the vaccine resulted in low uptake of the vaccine in Nigeria in the 1990s. Some Muslin leaders stated that the vaccine contained both antifertility drugs and the AIDS virus, and these caused sterilisation in children. Similar concerns emerged among Muslim groups in India, Pakistan and Afghanistan with refusals turning into waves of hostility 'and even cases of murder of the vaccinators'. Negotiations between faith leaders and health authorities, and visits from UNICEF and WHO, slowly restored some trust among some local communities. However, strong antivaccination sentiments persist in some regions of India and Pakistan [44, 45].

Another problem was cross-border transmission, in which the disease is spread to polio-free countries from areas that are still infected. Substantial movement of people between Afghanistan and Pakistan is spreading polio among under vaccinated communities. The Democratic Republic of Congo is another country with porous borders and as a result has experienced outbreaks of polio between 2021 and 2023. Poor sanitation, poverty and limited access to healthcare exacerbate disease spread [46, 47].

Possibly the most challenging problem first emerged during the elimination of polio in the Americas. The polio virus has a high mutation rate and is able to recombine (swaps bits of genetic material) with other polio viruses. These processes modified the strains of poliovirus used in the oral vaccine, producing variants that caused disease much like the original wild type virus. Most of these vaccine-derived strains were from the type 2 virus component of the vaccine [38, 48, 49].

In response the World Health Assembly recommended that the oral vaccine, which was active against all three types of polio, should be replaced by one that did not include type 2. This major change was implemented in 2016, with a type 2 inactivated vaccine to be used alongside the amended oral vaccine. Unfortunately the plan was less successful than hoped. Between 2016 and 2021 there were 2091 cases of polio. Most of these, 1727, were caused by the vaccine-derived type 2 virus, 91 by the two other types of vaccine-derived virus and 273 by wild type virus. The preponderance of cases of vaccine-derived type 2 virus is partly due to low vaccination coverage because of insufficient supplies of the inactivated type 2 vaccine. In addition, the inactivated vaccine is less effective at preventing transmission of the infection from person to person [49–51].

When Will Polio be Eradicated?

In theory polio eradication should be straightforward. Humans are the sole reservoir of the virus, and highly effective vaccines are available. But the story of polio vaccination is that major advances are interrupted by new outbreaks. The original target date was eradication by 2000, but this was successively postponed to 2004, 2008, 2012, 2018 and recently to 2026. During the eradication campaign about 20 million cases of paralytic polio have been prevented. In the process two of the wild types have been certified as eradicated: type 2 in 2015 and type 3 in 2019 [45, 52–54].

But problems remain. The type 1 wild type virus is still in circulation in Afghanistan and Pakistan, with case numbers fluctuating between 5 and 22 from 2021 to 2023. In the year to June 2024, vaccine-derived polio virus caused 74 outbreaks in 39 countries with vaccine-derived type 2 virus accounting for almost all of them. Local immunisation campaigns have only interrupted 11 of these outbreaks. Most telling is that in 2023, 12 cases of paralytic polio were caused by the type 1 wild type virus whereas 373 such cases were due to vaccine-derived virus (mainly type 2). A plan to prevent all outbreaks vaccine-derived virus in 2024 has failed. The intention to eradicate all new polio infections by 2026 seems unlikely to succeed [45, 53, 55].

There are signs that improved control of polio is possible. A new oral vaccine which targets type 2 virus but has a much lower likelihood of causing paralysis has been approved for mass distribution. Nearly one billion doses of this new vaccine had been administered by January 2024. Novel types of vaccine are also being developed which can reduce the manufacturing costs while ensuring safety and effectiveness. Further, improved surveillance methods are being used to identify and control new outbreaks [53, 55, 56].

The polio eradication programme relies on political commitment, support from local communities and continued funding. From the launch of the eradication campaign in 1988 over $20 billion has been spent on tackling polio. The annual spend was about $1.2 billion per year. Given the persistence of new outbreaks, current funding levels appear inadequate. As well as vaccine-derived virus, the present challenges include low vaccination coverage, suboptimal surveillance, armed conflicts, political instabilities and vaccine refusal. If these are not overcome, polio will remain a problem for many years to come [57, 58].

References

1. Hutchison, R. (1932). The medical history of sir Walter Scott. *Edinburgh Medical Journal, 39*(8), 461–485.
2. Drutz, J., & Ligon, B. (2000). Polio: Its history and its eradication. *Seminars in Pediatric Infectious Diseases, 11*, 280–286.
3. Varotto, E., Nizzo, V., & Galassi, F. M. (2019). Poliomyelitis in ancient Greece (5th century BC)? *Neurology, 92*(14), 678–679.
4. Cayton, E. (1989). The phenomenon of polio part I. From antiquity to the twenty-first century. *Baylor University Medical Center Proceedings, 2*(1), 5–14.
5. Paul, J. (1955). Epidemiology of poliomyelitis. In *Poliomyelitis. World Health Organization monograph series* (pp. 9–29). World Health Organization.
6. Trevelyan, B., Smallman-Raynor, M. R., & Cliff, A. (2005). The spatial dynamics of poliomyelitis in the United States: From epidemic emergence to vaccine-induced retreat, 1910–1971. *Annals of the Association of American Geographers, 95*, 269–293.
7. Robb, A. G. (1916). Recent epidemic outbreaks of acute poliomyelitis. *British Medical Journal, 2*(2905), 324–326.

8. Trevelyan, B., Smallman-Raynor, M., & Cliff, A. D. (2005). The spatial structure of epidemic emergence: Geographical aspects of poliomyelitis in North-Eastern USA, July-October 1916. *Journal of the Royal Statistical Society, Series A, 168*(4), 701–722.
9. Anonymous. (2016). The epidemic of infantile paralysis. *Journal of the American Medical Association, 316*(1), 107.
10. Nicoll, M. (1917). Epidemiological data in the poliomyelitis epidemic in New York state. *American Journal of Diseases of Children, 14*, 69–79.
11. Axelsson, P. (2009). "Do not eat those apples; they've been on the ground!": polio epidemics and preventive measures, Sweden 1880s-1940s. *Asclepio, 61*(1), 23–38.
12. Cockburn, W. C., & Drozdov, S. G. (1970). Poliomyelitis in the world. *Bulletin of the World Health Organization, 42*(3), 405–417.
13. Gear, J. (1955). Poliomyelitis in under-developed areas of the world. In *Poliomyelitis. World Health Organization monograph series*. World Health Organization.
14. Paul, J. R. (1954). Historical and geographical aspects of the epidemiology of poliomyelitis. *Yale Journal of Biology and Medicine, 27*(2), 101–113.
15. Caverly, C. (1896). Notes of an epidemic of acute anterior poliomyelitis. *JAMA, 26*, 1–4.
16. Collier, J. (1927). An address on the epidemiology and pathology of poliomyelitis. *British Medical Journal, 1*(3459), 751–753.
17. Eggers, H. J. (1999). Milestones in early poliomyelitis research (1840 to 1949). *Journal of Virology, 73*(6), 4533–4535.
18. Kramer, S. D. (1932). Experimental poliomyelitis: Its contribution to our knowledge of the human disease. *American Journal of Public Health and the Nation's Health, 22*(4), 381–390.
19. Melnick, J. L. (1996). Current status of poliovirus infections. *Clinical Microbiology Reviews, 9*(3), 293–300.
20. Alexander, J. P., Jr., Gary, H. E., Jr., & Pallansch, M. A. (1997). Duration of poliovirus excretion and its implications for acute flaccid paralysis surveillance: A review of the literature. *Journal of Infectious Diseases, 175*(Suppl 1), S176–S182.
21. Racaniello, V. R. (2006). One hundred years of poliovirus pathogenesis. *Virology, 344*(1), 9–16.
22. Bonville, C., & Suryadevara, M. (2021). Polio. In J. D. MS (Ed.), *Vaccine*. Springer Nature.

23. Pham, T., Brochard, L. J., & Slutsky, A. S. (2017). Mechanical ventilation: State of the art. *Mayo Clinic Proceedings, 92*(9), 1382–1400.
24. Trubuhovich, R. V. (2003). In the beginning. The 1952-1953 Danish epidemic of poliomyelitis and Bjørn Ibsen. *Critical Care and Resuscitation, 5*(3), 227–230.
25. Pichel, J. I. (1950). The age incidence of poliomyelitis in Connecticut, 1921-1947. *Yale Journal of Biology and Medicine, 22*(4), 327–340.
26. Nathanson, N., & Martin, J. R. (1979). The epidemiology of poliomyelitis: Enigmas surrounding its appearance, epidemicity, and disappearance. *American Journal of Epidemiology, 110*(6), 672–692.
27. Dauer, C. (1948). Trends in age distribution of poliomyelitis in the United States. *American Journal of Hygiene, 48*, 133–146.
28. Nelson, N. (1947). Present concepts of the epidemiology of poliomyelitis. *California Medicine, 67*(4), 224–226.
29. Nathanson, N., & Kew, O. M. (2010). From emergence to eradication: The epidemiology of poliomyelitis deconstructed. *American Journal of Epidemiology, 172*(11), 1213–1229.
30. Marks, H. M. (2011). The 1954 Salk poliomyelitis vaccine field trial. *Clinical Trials, 8*(2), 224–234.
31. Vashishtha, V. M., & Kamath, S. (2016). A brief history of vaccines against polio. *Indian Pediatrics, 53*(Suppl 1), S20–Ss7.
32. Orsini, D., & Martinin, M. (2022). Albert Bruce Sabin: The man who made the oral polio vaccine. *Emerging Infectious Diseases, 28*, 743–746.
33. Sabin, A. B. (1956). Pathogenesis of poliomyelitis; reappraisal in the light of new data. *Science, 123*(3209), 1151–1157.
34. Blume, S., & Geesink, I. (2000). A brief history of polio vaccines. *Science, 288*(5471), 1593–1594.
35. de Quadros, C. A., Andrus, J. K., Olive, J. M., Guerra de Macedo, C., & Henderson, D. A. (1992). Polio eradication from the Western hemisphere. *Annual Review of Public Health, 13*, 239–252.
36. Pedreira, C., Thrush, E., Rey-Benito, G., Chévez, A. E., & Jauregui, B. (2017). The path towards polio eradication over 40 years of the expanded program on immunization in the Americas. *Revista Panamericana de Salud Pública, 41*, e154.
37. Hampton, L. (2009). Albert Sabin and the coalition to eliminate polio from the Americas. *American Journal of Public Health, 99*(1), 34–44.
38. Nathanson, N. (1982). Eradication of poliomyelitis in the United States. *Reviews of Infectious Diseases, 4*(5), 940–950.

39. Hull, H. F., Ward, N. A., Hull, B. P., Milstien, J. B., & de Quadros, C. (1994). Paralytic poliomyelitis: Seasoned strategies, disappearing disease. *Lancet, 343*(8909), 1331–1337.
40. Anonymous. (2002). "Endgame" issues for the global polio eradication initiative. *Clinical Infectious Diseases, 34*(1), 72–77.
41. Aylward, B., & Tangermann, R. (2011). The global polio eradication initiative: Lessons learned and prospects for success. *Vaccine, 29*(Suppl 4), D80.
42. Jiang, B., Patel, M., & Glass, R. I. (2019). Polio endgame: Lessons for the global rotavirus vaccination program. *Vaccine, 37*(23), 3040–3049.
43. Beshr, I. A., Beshr, M. S., & Al-Qubati, H. A. (2023). Polio outbreak response, Yemen. *Bulletin of the World Health Organization, 101*(12), 808–812.
44. Agbede, G., Emezirinwune, D., Adedokun, T., et al. (2024). Vaccine hesitancy in Nigeria: Overcoming cultural, linguistic and religious obstacles. *Journal of Information and Knowledge, 15*, 153–168.
45. Seytre, B. (2023). Vaccine refusal: A major, underestimated obstacle for the poliomyelitis eradication initiative. *American Journal of Tropical Medicine and Hygiene, 109*(1), 6–9.
46. Sodhar, I. A., Mehraj, J., Hussaini, A. S., Aamir, M., Mahsaud, J., Ahmed, S., et al. (2024). Population movement and poliovirus spread across Pakistan and Afghanistan in 2023. *Vaccines (Basel)., 12*(9), 1006.
47. Oduoye, M. O., Ubechu, S. C., Mourid, M. R., Ahmad, A. I., Adegoke, A. A., Arama, U. O., et al. (2024). Re-emergence of vaccine-derived polio in the demographic republic of Congo: Causes and consequences. *New Microbes New Infections, 62*, 101489.
48. Savolainen-Kopra, C., & Blomqvist, S. (2010). Mechanisms of genetic variation in polioviruses. *Reviews in Medical Virology, 20*(6), 358–371.
49. Lai, Y. A., Chen, X., Kunasekaran, M., Rahman, B., & MacIntyre, C. R. (2022). Global epidemiology of vaccine-derived poliovirus 2016-2021: A descriptive analysis and retrospective case-control study. *EClinicalMedicine, 50*, 101508.
50. Macklin, G. R., O'Reilly, K. M., Grassly, N. C., Edmunds, W. J., Mach, O., Santhana Gopala Krishnan, R., et al. (2020). Evolving epidemiology of poliovirus serotype 2 following withdrawal of the serotype 2 oral poliovirus vaccine. *Science, 368*(6489), 401–405.
51. Sutter, R., Eisenhawer, M., Molodecky, N., Verma, H., & Okayasu, H. (2024). Inactivated poliovirus vaccine: Recent developments and the tortuous path to global acceptance. *Pathogens, 13*(3), 224.

52. Bigouette, J. P., Wilkinson, A. L., Tallis, G., Burns, C. C., Wassilak, S. G. F., & Vertefeuille, J. F. (2021). Progress toward polio eradication - worldwide, January 2019-June 2021. *Morbidity and Mortality Weekly Report, 70*(34), 1129–1135.
53. Lopez Cavestany, R., Eisenhawer, M., Diop, O. M., Verma, H., Quddus, A., & Mach, O. (2024). The last mile in polio eradication: Program challenges and perseverance. *Pathogens, 13*(4), 323.
54. Badizadegan, K., Kalkowska, D. A., & Thompson, K. M. (2022). Polio by the numbers-a global perspective. *Journal of Infectious Diseases, 226*(8), 1309–1318.
55. Burkholder, B., Wadood, Z., Kassem, A. M., Ehrhardt, D., & Zomahoun, D. (2023). The immediate impact of the COVID-19 pandemic on polio immunization and surveillance activities. *Vaccine, 41*(Suppl 1), A2–a11.
56. Kurji, F. D., Bandyopadhyay, A. S., Zipursky, S., Cooper, L. V., Gast, C., Toher, M., et al. (2024). Novel oral polio vaccine type 2 use for polio outbreak response: A global effort for a global health emergency. *Pathogens, 13*(4), 273.
57. Tediosi, F., Villa, S., Levison, D., Ekeman, E., & Politi, C. (2024). Leveraging global investments for polio eradication to strengthen health systems' resilience through transition. *Health Policy and Planning, 39*(Supplement_1), i93–i106.
58. Namageyo-Funa, A., Greene, S. A., Henderson, E., Traoré, M. A., Shaukat, S., Bigouette, J. P., et al. (2024). Update on vaccine-derived poliovirus outbreaks - worldwide, January 2023-June 2024. *Morbidity and Mortality Weekly Report, 73*(41), 909–916.

Measles

Measles is the most infectious of human diseases. On average each infected person will pass it on to about 12–18 other people. This high infectivity has ensured that the disease has been spread to every country in the world. It is easily recognised by the flattish small red spots that first appear on the face, although the white spots that appear on the inside of the cheeks are the real tell-tale sign of measles. The facial rash spreads gradually downwards from to cover the whole body, including the palms of the hands and soles of the feet. It disappears after 2–5 days. People who have had measles have lifelong immunity against subsequent infection [1, 2].

Measles in Children

Measles is often considered a relatively mild disease of children which has few complications. Those infected have a high fever, a cough, a runny or blocked nose and watery red eyes. The characteristic rash appears on the face and neck a few days after the symptoms begin. Nowadays most patients make a full recovery. But measles was once a major killer of infants older than 6 months. An Arabic proverb advises that parents

© The Author(s), under exclusive license to Springer Nature Singapore Pte Ltd. 2025

I. K Crombie, *Major Pandemics*, https://doi.org/10.1007/978-981-95-2081-7_9

should 'Count your children after the measles has passed'. In Parsee (the language of a large religious group in India) the proverb is more direct: 'Smallpox will make your child blind. Measles will send him to his grave' [3, 4].

Studies from 100 years ago provide confirmation of the folk wisdom on deaths in children. In Stockholm at the end of the nineteenth-century mortality rates from measles were high among children: some 60% of measles deaths occurred in children aged 3 months to 2 years. Mortality data from the State of New York in the early twentieth century confirms the finding that in children under 3 years of age measles is a dangerous disease: 70% of all deaths from measles occurred in this age group. This disease may be the worst killer of children the world has seen [5–7].

However, very young infants seldom contract measles. For the first 4–6 months of life, they are protected from infection by the maternal antibodies that cross through the placenta and are passed through breast milk. These antibodies gradually disappear as the infant's own immune system develops. By 6 months most infants have lost the early protection and are at risk of measles infection and its complications [8, 9].

Complications

Deaths from measles are usually caused by complications. Measles infection suppresses the body's immune response so that opportunistic bacteria and viruses can invade and cause serious illness. The most common of these complications are diarrhoea, pneumonia, croup and otitis media (infection of the middle ear). Pneumonia accounts for over half of the deaths following measles infection. Neurological complications are rare but usually serious. Almost all of the complications occur in children under 10 years of age, with children less than 12 months being at highest risk. Modern antibiotics can resolve most of the secondary bacterial infections and vitamin A supplementation during acute measles can significantly reduce the death rate. The frequency of complications has fallen substantially in high-income countries, but remains high in many low- and middle-income countries [8, 10, 11].

Origin of Measles

Measles is descended from rinderpest, an ancient virus that infected cattle and other animals such as goats, camels, pigs, deer, giraffes and wildebeest. The term 'rinderpest' comes from a German word meaning cattle-plague. This disease may have originated in Asia, at the time when cattle were first domesticated some 10,000 years ago. It was probably introduced into Europe in the Middle Ages by invading armies from the east [12].

Molecular studies suggest that the measles virus diverged from rinderpest and made the leap from animals into humans about 2500 years ago. This was the time when humans began to gather together in large towns and cities. That is important as measles needs large populations to survive. Because it is highly infectious, all the people in small settlements would quickly contract the disease and become immune to further infection. The virus would become extinct because there was no one left to infect. It was only with the emergence of large towns and cities that measles could be sustained in a community. Populations of at least 250,000 people are needed to maintain measles infections [13, 14].

How Measles Spreads

The disease is contracted by being close to an infected person who coughs or sneezes, spraying virus-laden droplets and aerosols into the air. While airborne, the virus remains active for up to 2 h, so that people nearby can be infected. As most cases are infectious from 4 days before to 4 days after the rash appears, many people can be exposed to an infectious individual without realising it. Only a low dose of virus is needed to cause infection, so anyone not previously infected is likely to contract the disease [3, 15, 16].

The measles virus is well adapted to be spread in human populations. When the measles-laden droplets and aerosols are inhaled, the virus binds to specific receptors on cells in the lungs. These cells (dendritic cells and lymphocytes) are part of the body's immune response system. The virus employs several mechanisms that allow it to avoid being destroyed by these cells. Instead, it replicates in them. Some of the infected immune cells carry the virus around the body to the gastrointestinal tract, kidney, liver, skin and, less commonly, the central nervous system. The virus then uses other receptors to infect the cells of these organs. Finally, the virus uses a different receptor to infect and destroy cells lining the lungs. This causes the patient to cough violently, completing the cycle of transmission [16–18].

Isolated Communities

The infectiousness of measles is most clearly seen when the disease enters an isolated community for the first time. Up until 1874 the islands of Fiji had never suffered an outbreak. Then in September 1874, a delegation led by chief Cokabau visited Sydney to sign a treaty making the Fijian islands a protectorate of the British Empire. While in Australia they must have been exposed to measles because on their return to Fiji on 12 January, two of the chief's sons became ill with the disease. Once back home a gathering of the prominent hill chiefs was held on 24 January to discuss/celebrate Fiji's new status as a protectorate. Unfortunately many of the participants contracted measles and carried it with them when they returned home. When a quarantine was imposed on 25 February to prevent the transmission to the other islands, it was too late. The virus was widely spread through the Fijian islands. Somewhere between 20,000 and 50,000 people died out of a population of about 120,000. The mortality may have been high because in each village most people became ill at the same time, so they were unable to procure and cook food for each other. The epidemic ended in June 1875, when almost everyone had been infected with measles [19, 20].

A more recent example is the 1951 outbreak in southern Greenland, an isolated region that had no experience of measles. The outbreak began when a young sailor, who had recently returned from Denmark, attended a dance. He was subsequently admitted to hospital where he was diagnosed with measles. Within 3 months, 99.9% of the population of 4320 people had been infected. A similar high rate of infection occurred in a community of Indians and Eskimos living in Canada's Arctic Circle in

1952. In this outbreak 99% of the population were infected and 7% died [21, 22].

Some isolated communities have an outbreak of measles and then, many years later, suffer a second one. This happened to the Faroes, a group of islands that are halfway between the UK and Iceland. Measles was most likely transported by a cabinet maker who travelled from Copenhagen and arrived in Tórshavn, the capital city of the Faroes, on 28 March 1846. A few days later he developed symptoms of measles. A young doctor, Peter Ludwig Panum, was sent by the Danish Government to investigate the outbreak. He showed that only people under the age of 65 caught the infection. There had been a previous outbreak of measles in 1781, and those who contracted the disease then were immune to the 1846 outbreak [23, 24].

Periodic Outbreaks

Until the 1960s countries with more than a million inhabitants had regular outbreaks of infection. These took the form of a very rapid increase in cases followed by an equally swift decline. For example, over the period 1950–1968, England and Wales experienced regular large spikes in 1 year, which were followed by equally large troughs the following year. This periodicity is a long-standing phenomenon; data on deaths in London from 1703 to 1912 show peaks every second year. A similar pattern was seen for New York City between 1928 and 1962, although the interval between the peaks is less regular. In Denmark between 1946 and 1974 the interval was 2.5 years. The time between spikes tends to be longer in countries with comparatively sparse population. For example, data from Australia between 1890 and 1905 show regular peaks of infection with an interval of 5 years. In Sweden in the eighteenth and nineteenth centuries the gap between spikes was even longer at 6 years [25–30].

The regularity of outbreaks occurs because measles is highly infectious, and infection confers lifelong immunity. When measles first enters a country, most people are infected and for a few years no new outbreaks can occur. But the number of susceptible individuals will increase as new babies are born and non-immune people migrate into the country. When the number of immune people falls below a threshold then a new outbreak will occur. The threshold for measles is about 95%. When less than 95% of the population are immune, there will be a spike in the number of new cases. As the outbreak continues and more people become infected, the threshold is exceeded and the number of cases rapidly falls [3].

The Early History

The history of measles is obscure because the early physicians and scholars did not distinguish it from other diseases which caused rashes, particularly smallpox. The first clinical description was provided by Abu Bakr Muhammad Ibn Zakariya al-Razi, a Persian scholar and physician who lived from 865 to 925 BCE. (He was known in Western medicine as Rhazes.) Among many other achievements in medicine, he distinguished measles from smallpox. He also recommended staying well away from patients in the early stages of infection to prevent the disease from spreading [31].

The term 'measles' first appears in English in 1325 when it was written as maselys. It may have derived from the Dutch word *masela* or the German words *maes* or *mas* meaning a spot. Maselys was used to describe anyone with skin eruptions or sores. In European medicine the use of measles as a catch-all term for a disease with spots persisted until the seventeenth century when greater emphasis was placed on the precise diagnosis [32, 33].

Like other diseases that have plagued humans for centuries, many explanations have been offered for the onset of measles. Astrological phenomena were commonly invoked to explain disease outbreaks, with the planets Mars and Venus being accused of emitting deadly exhalations that spread measles infection. In seventeenth-century Europe, mothers were often blamed for inflicting the disease on their children. The theory was that when a woman stopped menstruating during pregnancy, her blood became contaminated and the impurities were passed to the growing foetus. This corrupted menstrual blood caused the fever and the rash of spots. Another suggestion is that breast milk curdled into acid, creating impurities in the blood of the suckling child. In Africa, sorcery, or foodstuffs such as snails, were thought to cause measles, whereas in Asia a malignant goddess was blamed [4, 34].

Global Spread

From its origin some 2500 years ago, measles was thought to have spread across most of Asia and all of Europe by the Middle Ages. The subsequent spread around the world began in the sixteenth century with the Spanish in their conquests of Central and South America. The success of a few hundred soldiers, led by men such as Cortez and Pizarro, in defeating much larger armies was in large part due to infectious diseases, particularly smallpox but also measles. It is likely that European colonial expansion in the seventeenth century carried measles to much of the rest of the world. However, it did not arrive in Australia until the 1850s [31].

Measles has probably been a cause of disease and death in Africa for hundreds of years, but the evidence for this is exceedingly sparse. A report from Ghana in the mid-1800s suggests that the infection was common and often fatal in young children. The disease was also widespread across India at this time with outbreaks in many regions occurring almost every year [35, 36].

Measles in the First Half of the Twentieth Century

In the industrialised countries, death rates from measles fell progressively from the end of the nineteenth century. From 1850 to 1890 in England and Wales, the death rate was constant at about 40 per 100,000 people. Then it fell slowly to 30 per 100,000 in 1905, then more quickly to 6 per 100,000 in 1921 reaching 0.4 per 100,000 in 1961. Data from the United States and Italy show a similar steady fall in death rates through the first six decades of the twentieth century. But the data from the United States also show that, although the number of deaths fell, the number of cases remained broadly constant. Clearly infection was still widespread, but fewer people were dying [37–39].

The substantial falls in mortality were most likely due to a combination of improved nutrition, better housing and reduced overcrowding. Most other infectious disease, such as tuberculosis, whooping cough, scarlet fever and diphtheria, showed similar declines in mortality from the end of the nineteenth century through to the middle of the twentieth. Improvements in general standards of living are the most likely explanation for the reductions in mortality rates of all these diseases [39–41].

Low- and Middle-Income Countries

Data on the frequency of cases and deaths from measles in low- and middle-income countries in the first half of the twentieth century are sparse. What is clear is that the disease was common in all except the most isolated communities. In the mid-1900s measles was a common disease in Africa, and feared because of the high mortality in children under five. South America, India and much of Asia also suffered from measles [4, 35, 42].

The Vaccine

The development of an effective vaccine against measles in the 1960s dramatically reduced both cases and deaths from measles. The measles virus was first isolated in 1954, and research to develop a vaccine began shortly after. Two types of vaccine for measles were developed in the 1950s. One of them used inactivated (killed) virus, but the level of immunity it induced quickly faded. Children given this vaccine were also at risk developing an unpleasant and atypical form of measles if exposed to an infected person. This vaccine was subsequently abandoned. The other type of vaccine used a live virus that had been attenuated (weakened) by being repeatedly grown in cells in the laboratory. It induced high levels of immunity, but also caused a rash and a fever. This side effect was overcome by further rounds of attenuation in laboratory cells, to yield a highly effective vaccine with few side effects. To achieve maximum benefit the vaccine is administered to young children in two doses: the first at 9–12 months and the next between 2 and 5 years of age [43, 44].

The live attenuated vaccine was licensed for use in 1963 and the United States took the lead by beginning a mass immunisation campaign. Its impact was dramatic. Numbers of cases in the United States fell from over 400,000 per year in 1963 to less than 50,000 3 years later. The reduction continued so that by the year 2000 there were less than 100 cases a year. The early success of this initiative led to a concerted campaign in North and South America that eliminated measles from the whole region by 2002 [45, 46].

In Europe, the view that measles infection was a normal part of childhood led to a more cautious approach to mass vaccination. The UK measles vaccination programme only began in 1968. Initially coverage was low, about 30%, but slowly increased to 63% among children under two by 1983. Then in 1988 a national campaign was implemented targeting all young children combined with a catch-up for school-age children. This increased the vaccination rate to just over 90% by the early 1990s [47, 48].

This pattern was largely replicated across in Europe. In 1980 only 63% of children had been vaccinated by 12 months of age. Finland successfully managed to immunise >95% of its population with two doses of vaccine in 1994. At that time only a few countries in the region, such as the Netherlands, Poland and Portugal, achieved vaccination coverage above 90%. Several countries, for example Ireland, Greece and Germany, achieved less than 80% coverage [49, 50].

The MMR Vaccine

A combined measles, mumps and rubella vaccine (MMR) was adopted in the 1970s in the United States, in Britain in 1988. It was also included in the World Health Organization's expanded programme on immunisation. This combined vaccine saves repeated visits to a doctor, increasing the uptake of immunisation against all three diseases. But trouble came in 1998 when a report by Wakefield and colleagues was published in a leading medical journal. It suggested that the MMR vaccine could cause autism in children. The claim, which was subsequently shown to be completely false, generated substantial media coverage and led to a dramatic reduction in the uptake of the vaccine in Britain. The uptake of vaccination fell over the next few years, and the number of cases of measles increased from <100 in the late 1990s to over 2000 in 2012. Similar falls in vaccination rates led to increases in cases across Europe and the United States. With the public disgrace of Wakefield, and compelling evidence that the MMR vaccine does not cause autism, immunisation rates increased. However in many countries the rates are lower than they were before the Wakefield debacle [51–53].

Expanding Coverage in Low- and Middle-Income Countries

In the 1960s measles death rates of children in most low- and middle-income countries were appallingly high. At that time in the UK about 20 per 100,000 children with measles died, whereas in less advantaged countries the figure was 2000 per 100,000. To reduce these high death rates the World Health Organization launched its Expanded Programme of Immunization in 1974. Measles was added to the global immunisation programmes for the other vaccine preventable diseases (polio, tetanus, tuberculosis, diphtheria, whooping cough). The initial phase aimed at vaccinating 80% of children aged 9 months in every country of the world. The second phase introduced a second dose for children entering primary school to ensure coverage of those who did not gain immunity after the first dose. The Expanded Programme of Immunization campaign has had a substantial impact on measles infections. Prior to the campaign there were an estimated 106 million cases of measles and 5.7 million deaths each year. By 1995, these had fallen to 26.5 million cases and 780,000 deaths. But because immunisation rates had stagnated at 70–80%, a third phase was implemented in the year 2000. It targeted the 45 countries that accounted for 90% of global deaths from measles. This phase aimed to achieve vaccination levels above 90% and to reduce by 50% the number of deaths [54–56].

Supplementary Immunisation Activities

Programmes of Supplementary Immunisation Activities (SIA) were introduced to boost vaccination rates in children living in areas which were falling far short of the target of 95% coverage with two doses of vaccine. They were widely implemented in the Americas in the 1990s as part of a strategy to eradicate measles in that region by 2002. In other regions they were targeted at children in areas with low vaccination coverage, including those that are hard to reach [57, 58].

Global Trends from 2000

In the year 2000 a total of 853,479 of measles were reported to the World Health Organization. The numbers fell progressively to a minimum of 132,000 cases in 2016 before climbing back to 873,000 in 2019. The data on reported cases from 2020 to 2022 are unreliable because the Covid-19 pandemic seriously impaired the identification and reporting of new cases of measles. The reported number of global cases fell to 60,000 in 2021. Since then, case numbers have risen again to reach just over 660,000 by 2023. It is unclear how much of this is due a gradual recovery in case reporting and how much to a real increase in the rate of infection [59, 60].

Because most cases of infection are not reported, researchers have used modelling techniques to estimate the total number of infections. This showed that there were just over 36.9 million cases in 2000, and this had reduced to 10.3 million cases in 2023. Over that period the estimated deaths fell from 200,000 to 107,500 in 2023 [60].

Global vaccination coverage with the first dose rose from 71% in 2000 to 83% in 2023, but the number of countries who reached the 95% threshold only increased from 28 to 35 (from a total of 194). From a very low base of 17% in 2000, coverage with second dose shot up to 74% in 2023, but is still far short of the 95% target. Between 2022 and 2023 many countries in Africa, the Western Pacific, South East Asia, the Eastern Mediterranean and Europe experienced many 'large or disruptive outbreaks' of measles. This is probably due to vaccination levels below the 95% threshold [60].

When Will it End

In theory measles is an ideal disease for eradication. Several features indicate that this it is biologically, technically and operationally possible. Humans are the only reservoir of infection. The vaccine is highly effective and provides long-lasting immunity, and the virus does not mutate to escape the immunity given by immunisation. Accurate and rapid diagnostic tests had been developed so that any outbreaks could be identified quickly, enabling supplementary immunisation to be implemented. Finally, the economic gains of eradication are substantial. The costs of treating those who become ill and the productivity lost because of illness, disabled or death greatly outweigh the costs of delivering the vaccination programme. In low- and middle-income countries, which suffer the major burden of infection, the benefits of vaccination outweigh the costs by a factor of 16 to 1 [61, 62].

The United States pioneered mass vaccination campaigns so that the whole of the Americas had eradicated measles by 2002. This achievement kindled hopes of the global elimination of measles. Because measles is very infectious, high levels of immunity are needed to prevent ongoing spread. Vaccination levels that fall short of the recommended 95% will not only lead to measles outbreaks in low-coverage regions, but, given high volumes of air travel, it will lead to international spread of infection. As Durrheim and colleagues remarked, 'measles anywhere is a problem everywhere'. Even the United States is still troubled by imported measles: between 2020 and 2024 almost all of 338 cases had come from other countries [63, 64].

The high-income countries have largely controlled measles through the combination of greatly improved living standards and high levels of vaccination. In contrast many low- and middle-income countries have to contend with overcrowding, the ideal condition for high intensity of measles transmission. Low levels of dietary vitamin A increase also increase the risk that children will die from measles [65].

Another problem is vaccine hesitancy. This covers a wide range of attitudes, from uncertainty about vaccination to outright hostility towards the process. People in every country have concerns about the safety and efficacy of vaccines, but there is substantial variation between them. Some countries, such as Italy, France and Russia, have least confidence in vaccines, whereas countries in Africa and South America have much higher levels of confidence. Vaccine hesitancy is being fuelled by anti-vax activists who spread misleading messages on social media. These claim that vaccines are ineffective and harmful and that there is a conspiracy to thrust them onto an unsuspecting public. The United States has particularly vigorous activists who are successfully disrupting vaccination programmes. Vaccine hesitancy affects immunisation campaigns in over 90% of countries. Common reasons were fear of side effects, lack of knowledge of the benefits and a conflict with traditional cultural beliefs. Influential leaders, concerns about the organisation and delivery of the vaccine programmes and both anti- and pro-vaccination lobbies also affected uptake [66–69].

In summary, remarkable progress has been made in controlling measles infections. But with global vaccination rates remaining consistently below the target of 95% and over 10 million cases and 100,000 deaths each year, the ending of the pandemic is many years away. If substantial extra financial support could be found, supported by the firm commitment of political leaders, great progress could be made. But that would still leave the challenge of the end game, where a few hundreds of cases can continue to seed new outbreaks. The experience of polio eradication has shown how difficult it is to eradicate a disease. In 1988 the aim was to do this by the year 2000, but 25 years later the world was still struggling with the last few hundred cases of polio. Given its much higher infectivity, ending the measles pandemic is likely to be a much more difficult task [59, 70, 71].

References

1. Battegay, R., Itin, C., & Itin, P. (2012). Dermatological signs and symptoms of measles: a prospective case series and comparison with the literature. *Dermatology, 224*(1), 1–4.
2. Rota, P. A., Moss, W. J., Takeda, M., de Swart, R. L., Thompson, K. M., & Goodson, J. L. (2016). Measles. *Nature Reviews Disease Primers, 2*, 16049.
3. Guerra, F. M., Bolotin, S., Lim, G., Heffernan, J., Deeks, S. L., Li, Y., et al. (2017). The basic reproduction number (R(0)) of measles: A systematic review. *Lancet Infectious Diseases, 17*(12), e420–e428.
4. Morley, D. (1969). Severe measles in the tropics. I. *British Medical Journal, 1*(5639), 297–300. contd.
5. Burström, B., Diderichsen, F., Bernhardt, E., & Smedman, L. (1998). Use of a historical register in social epidemiology: Child mortality in Stockholm at the turn of the 19th century. *Scandinavian Journal of Social Medicine, 26*(3), 166–172.
6. Godfrey, E. S. (1926). The administrative control of measles. *American Journal of Public Health, 16*(6), 571–577.
7. Clements, C., & Hussey, G. (2004). Measles. In C. J. Murray & C. Mather (Eds.), *The global epidemiology of infectious diseases. Global burden of disease and injury series. IV* (pp. 75–110). World Health Organization.
8. Bester, J. C. (2016). Measles and measles vaccination: A review. *JAMA Pediatrics, 170*(12), 1209–1215.
9. Leuridan, E., & Van Damme, P. (2007). Passive transmission and persistence of naturally acquired or vaccine-induced maternal antibodies against measles in newborns. *Vaccine, 25*(34), 6296–6304.
10. Miller, D. L. (1964). The public health importance of measles in britain today. *Proceedings of the Royal Society of Medicine, 57*(9), 843–846.
11. Perry, R. T., & Halsey, N. A. (2004). The clinical significance of measles: A review. *Journal of Infectious Diseases, 189*(Suppl 1), S4–S16.
12. Roeder, P., Mariner, J., & Kock, R. (2013). Rinderpest: The veterinary perspective on eradication. *Philosophical Transactions of the Royal Society, B: Biological Sciences, 368*(1623), 20120139.
13. Düx, A., Lequime, S., Patrono, L. V., Vrancken, B., Boral, S., Gogarten, J. F., et al. (2020). Measles virus and rinderpest virus divergence dated to the sixth century BCE. *Science, 368*(6497), 1367–1370.
14. Keeling, M. J., & Grenfell, B. T. (1997). Disease extinction and community size: Modeling the persistence of measles. *Science, 275*(5296), 65–67.

15. World Health Organisation. (2024). *Measles: Key facts*. World Health Organisation. https://www.who.int/news-room/fact-sheets/detail/measles#:~:text=Transmission,for%20up%20to%20two%20hours
16. Hübschen, J. M., Gouandjika-Vasilache, I., & Dina, J. (2022). Measles. *Lancet, 399*(10325), 678–690.
17. Laksono, B. M., de Vries, R. D., McQuaid, S., Duprex, W. P., & de Swart, R. L. (2016). Measles virus host invasion and pathogenesis. *Viruses, 8*(8), 210.
18. Amurri, L., Reynard, O., Gerlier, D., Horvat, B., & Iampietro, M. (2022). Measles virus-induced host immunity and mechanisms of viral evasion. *Viruses, 14*(12), 2641.
19. Squire, W. (1879). On measles in Fiji. *Transactions of the Epidemiological Society of London, 4*(Pt 1), 72–74.
20. Morens, D. M. (1998). Measles in Fiji: Thoughts on the history of emerging infectious diseases. *Pacific Health Dialog, 5*, 119–128.
21. Christensen, P., Schmidt, H., Jensen, O., et al. (1953). An epidemic of measles in southern Greenland, 1951 Measles in virgin soil. *Acta Medica Scandinavica, 144*, 313–322.
22. Peart, A. F., & Nagler, F. P. (1954). Measles in the Canadian Arctic, 1952. *Canadian Journal of Public Health, 45*(4), 146–156.
23. Little, J. (1931). Peter Ludwig Panum 1820-1885: A pioneer in the epidemiology of measles. *Canadian Journal of Public Health, 22*, 509–516.
24. Klass, P., & Ratner, A. J. (2022). "The sombre aspect of the entire landscape" - Epidemiology and The Faroe Islands. *New England Journal of Medicine, 386*(13), 1202–1205.
25. Fine, P. E., & Clarkson, J. A. (1982). Measles in England and Wales—I: An analysis of factors underlying seasonal patterns. *International Journal of Epidemiology, 11*(1), 5–14.
26. Brownlee, J. (1918). An investigation into the periodicity of measles epidemics London from 1703 to the present day by the method of the periodogram. *Philosophical Transactions of the Royal Society B, 206*, 225–250.
27. London, W. P., & Yorke, J. A. (1973). Recurrent outbreaks of measles, chickenpox and mumps. I. Seasonal variation in contact rates. *American Journal of Epidemiology, 98*(6), 453–468.
28. Edmunds, W. J., Gay, N. J., Kretzschmar, M., Pebody, R. G., & Wachmann, H. (2000). The pre-vaccination epidemiology of measles, mumps and rubella in Europe: Implications for modelling studies. *Epidemiology and Infection, 125*(3), 635–650.

29. Ransome, A. (1883). On the form of the epidemic wave and some of its probable causes. *Transactions of the Epidemiological Society of London, 1*, 96–107.
30. Shanks, G. D., Waller, M., Briem, H., & Gottfredsson, M. (2015). Age-specific measles mortality during the late 19th-early 20th centuries. *Epidemiology and Infection, 143*(16), 3434–3441.
31. Berche, P. (2022). History of measles. *La Presse Médicale, 51*, 104149.
32. Sykes, W. (1896). On the origin and history of some disease names. *Lancet, 1*(3789), 1007–1010.
33. Brincker, J. A. (1938). A historical, epidemiological and aetiological study of measles (morbilli; rubeola): (section of epidemiology and state medicine). *Proceedings of the Royal Society of Medicine, 31*(7), 807–828.
34. Radbill, S. X., & Hamilton, G. R. (1960). Measles in fact and fancy. *Bulletin of the History of Medicine, 34*, 430–442.
35. Morley, D. (1964). The severe measles of West Africa. *Proceedings of the Royal Society of Medicine, 57*(9), 846–849.
36. Milroy, G. (1865). Notes on the epidemic and other diseases of the natives of India. *Transactions of the Epidemiological Society of London, 2*(Pt 1), 150–159.
37. Langmuir, A. D., Henderson, D. A., Serfling, R. E., & Sherman, I. L. (1962). The importance of measles as a health problem. *American Journal of Public Health and the Nation's Health, 52*(2), 1–4.
38. Logan, W. (1950). Mortality in England and Wales from 1848 to 1947. *Population Studies, 4*, 132–178.
39. Pezzotti, P., Bellino, S., Prestinaci, F., Iacchini, S., Lucaroni, F., Camoni, L., et al. (2018). The impact of immunization programs on 10 vaccine preventable diseases in Italy: 1900-2015. *Vaccine, 36*(11), 1435–1443.
40. Nieburg, P., & Dibley, M. J. (1986). Risk factors for fatal measles infections. *International Journal of Epidemiology, 15*(3), 309–311.
41. McKeown, T., Record, R. G., & Turner, R. D. (1975). An interpretation of the decline of mortality in England and Wales during the twentieth century. *Population Studies, 29*(3), 391–422.
42. World Health Organization. (1946). *Cases and deaths of measles reported in Europe and in certain countries outside Europe, 1928–1938 (medians) and 1944–1946.* World Health Organization. https://iris.who.int/bitstream/handle/10665/237980/WER2119_152-154.PDF
43. Griffin, D. E. (2018). Measles vaccine. *Viral Immunology, 31*(2), 86–95.

44. Hendriks, J., & Blume, S. (2013). Measles vaccination before the measles-mumps-rubella vaccine. *American Journal of Public Health, 103*(8), 1393–1401.
45. Strebel, P. M., & Orenstein, W. A. (2019). Measles. *New England Journal of Medicine, 381*(4), 349–357.
46. Castillo-Solorzano, C., Marsigli, C., Danovaro-Holliday, M. C., Ruiz-Matus, C., Tambini, G., & Andrus, J. K. (2011). Measles and rubella elimination initiatives in the Americas: Lessons learned and best practices. *Journal of Infectious Diseases, 204*(Suppl 1), S279–S283.
47. Noah, N. D. (1984). What can we do about measles? *British Medical Journal (Clinical Research Edition), 289*(6457), 1476.
48. Nokes, D. J., Williams, J. R., & Butler, A. R. (1995). Towards eradication of measles virus: global progress and strategy evaluation. *Veterinary Microbiology, 44*(2–4), 333–350.
49. Peltola, H., Heinonen, O. P., Valle, M., Paunio, M., Virtanen, M., Karanko, V., et al. (1994). The elimination of indigenous measles, mumps, and rubella from Finland by a 12-year, two-dose vaccination program. *New England Journal of Medicine, 331*(21), 1397–1402.
50. Asaria, P., & MacMahon, E. (2006). Measles in the United Kingdom: Can we eradicate it by 2010? *BMJ, 333*(7574), 890–895.
51. Tannous, L. K., Barlow, G., & Metcalfe, N. H. (2014). A short clinical review of vaccination against measles. *JRSM Open, 5*(4), 2054270414523408.
52. Carrillo-Santisteve, P., & Lopalco, P. L. (2012). Measles still spreads in Europe: who is responsible for the failure to vaccinate? *Clinical Microbiology and Infection, 18*(Suppl 5), 50–56.
53. DeStefano, F., & Shimabukuro, T. (2019). The MMR vaccine and autism. *Annual Review of Virology, 6*(1), 585–600.
54. Wolfson, L. J., Grais, R. F., Luquero, F. J., Birmingham, M. E., & Strebel, P. M. (2009). Estimates of measles case fatality ratios: A comprehensive review of community-based studies. *International Journal of Epidemiology, 38*(1), 192–205.
55. Henderson, R. H. (1984). The expanded programme on immunization of the World Health Organization. *Reviews of Infectious Diseases, 6*(Suppl 2), S475–S479.
56. Global Programme for Vaccines and Immunization. (1996). *Progress of vaccine research and development and plan of activities, 1996*. Global Programme for Vaccines and Immunization.

57. Auzenbergs, M., Fu, H., Abbas, K., Procter, S. R., Cutts, F. T., & Jit, M. (2023). Health effects of routine measles vaccination and supplementary immunisation activities in 14 high-burden countries: A dynamic measles immunization calculation engine (DynaMICE) modelling study. *The Lancet Global Health, 11*(8), e1194–e1204.
58. Portnoy, A., Jit, M., Helleringer, S., & Verguet, S. (2018). Impact of measles supplementary immunization activities on reaching children missed by routine programs. *Vaccine, 36*(1), 170–178.
59. Minta, A. A., Ferrari, M., Antoni, S., Portnoy, A., Sbarra, A., Lambert, B., et al. (2022). Progress toward regional measles elimination - worldwide, 2000-2021. *Morbidity and Mortality Weekly Report, 71*(47), 1489–1495.
60. Minta, A. A., Ferrari, M., Antoni, S., Lambert, B., Sayi, T. S., Hsu, C. H., et al. (2024). Progress toward measles elimination - worldwide, 2000-2023. *Morbidity and Mortality Weekly Report, 73*(45), 1036–1042.
61. Cochi, S. L., & Schluter, W. W. (2020). What it will take to achieve a world without measles. *Journal of Infectious Diseases, 222*(7), 1073–1075.
62. Ozawa, S., Clark, S., Portnoy, A., Grewal, S., Brenzel, L., & Walker, D. G. (2016). Return on investment from childhood immunization in low- and middle-income countries, 2011-20. *Health affairs (Project Hope), 35*(2), 199–207.
63. Durrheim, D. N. (2020). Measles eradication-retreating is not an option. *The Lancet Infectious Diseases, 20*(6), e138–e141.
64. Mathis, A. D., Raines, K., Masters, N. B., Filardo, T. D., Kim, G., Crooke, S. N., et al. (2024). Measles - United States, January 1, 2020-march 28, 2024. *Morbidity and Mortality Weekly Report, 73*(14), 295–300.
65. Black, R. E., Allen, L. H., Bhutta, Z. A., Caulfield, L. E., de Onis, M., Ezzati, M., et al. (2008). Maternal and child undernutrition: global and regional exposures and health consequences. *Lancet, 371*(9608), 243–260.
66. Dubé, E., Vivion, M., & MacDonald, N. E. (2015). Vaccine hesitancy, vaccine refusal and the anti-vaccine movement: influence, impact and implications. *Expert Review of Vaccines, 14*(1), 99–117.
67. Larson, H. J., de Figueiredo, A., Xiahong, Z., Schulz, W. S., Verger, P., Johnston, I. G., et al. (2016). The state of vaccine confidence 2016: Global insights through a 67-country survey. *eBioMedicine, 12*, 295–301.
68. Hotez, P. J., Nuzhath, T., & Colwell, B. (2020). Combating vaccine hesitancy and other 21st century social determinants in the global fight against measles. *Current Opinion in Virology, 41*, 1–7.

69. Lane, S., MacDonald, N. E., Marti, M., & Dumolard, L. (2018). Vaccine hesitancy around the globe: Analysis of three years of WHO/UNICEF joint reporting form data-2015-2017. *Vaccine, 36*(26), 3861–3867.
70. Patel, M. K., Goodson, J. L., Alexander, J. P., Jr., Kretsinger, K., Sodha, S. V., Steulet, C., et al. (2020). Progress toward regional measles elimination - worldwide, 2000-2019. *Morbidity and Mortality Weekly Report, 69*(45), 1700–1705.
71. Lopez Cavestany, R., Eisenhawer, M., Diop, O. M., Verma, H., Quddus, A., & Mach, O. (2024). The last mile in polio eradication: Program challenges and perseverance. *Pathogens, 13*(4), 323.

Tuberculosis

Introduction

Tuberculosis (TB) is one of the most deadly of infectious diseases. It has been given many names. The ancient Greeks called it *phthisis*, which meant to waste away. The father of modern medicine, Hippocrates (460–370 BCE), described it as a weakness of the lung with fever and cough almost always leading to death. *Consumption* was another term for TB. It indicated that the individual was consumed from within as the flesh rotted away. In the eighteenth century it was thought that there was a build-up of putrid blood in the lungs which caused the corrosion of other organs by ulcerous pus, leading to emaciation of the body. Although in no way accurate, this imagery correctly conveys a process of decay leading to death. In the nineteenth century the disease was given more descriptive names: the *robber of youth*, the *graveyard cough*, the *white plague* or the *white death*. These reflect the symptoms of the disease, particularly the paleness of the skin in the final stages of the illness. The wasting away and the change in skin colour were captured in a line from John Keats' poem 'Ode to a Nightingale': 'Where youth grows pale and spectre-thin and dies'. Keats died from TB shortly after writing it; he was

© The Author(s), under exclusive license to Springer Nature Singapore Pte Ltd. 2025

I. K Crombie, *Major Pandemics*, https://doi.org/10.1007/978-981-95-2081-7_10

only 25. The modern term *tuberculosis* was introduced in the mid-nineteenth century [1, 2].

The Nature of the Disease

Tuberculosis is caused by the bacterium *Mycobacterium tuberculosis* (*M. tuberculosis*). It was successfully identified by the acclaimed German scientist Robert Koch. He also discovered the bacteria that caused anthrax and cholera, and developed several important microbiological techniques while doing so. Koch was awarded the Nobel Prize for physiology and medicine in 1905, primarily for his work on TB [3].

M. tuberculosis usually attacks the lungs, producing symptoms of fever, fatigue, lack of appetite, weight loss, shortness of breath and a chronic cough that brings up a thick mucus. A cough that produces blood is a sign of serious disease. TB can be cured with a course of antibiotics, but if untreated about 70% of cases die within 3 years of disease onset [4, 5].

Many cases of TB only involve the lungs, but the bacterium can drain through the lymphatic system into the bloodstream, where it can infect other organs. Between 20% and 50% of cases present with infection outside the lung. A common form of this is the swelling of the lymph nodes in the neck. It was called the King's Evil, or scrofula, and caused painful, weeping sores. In England, from the time of Edward the Confessor in the eleventh century, people believed that the King could heal this disease by laying hands on the site of the illness. As scrofula can undergo spontaneous remission, the king's touch often appeared to cure the disease. The most diligent of the monarchs was Charles II, who is said to have touched some 100,000 scrofulous individuals during his reign [6, 7].

The other sites that can be infected include the bones and joints, the urinogenital system and the digestive system. Most commonly only one organ is attacked, but, in about 2% of cases, the bacterium spreads to multiple sites throughout the body causing what is called miliary TB. This is a particularly serious which, because several organs fail at the same time. All patients die without treatment [6, 8].

Based on data from screening tests, an estimated one-quarter of the world's population have been infected with *M. tuberculosis* but do not have any symptoms of the disease. This has been described as latent infection, in which the bacterium lay dormant in a quiet corner of the lungs. It was thought that the disease could be reactivated, particularly when the host immune system is compromised. With two billion people having latent infections, this became a major concern. However, more recent research has shown that most people who test positive for TB have cleared the bacterium from their bodies. What remains is an immunological memory of the infection, which would enable the body to respond quickly if re-infection occurred. Only a small proportion, 5–10%, of people with a previous infection go on to develop active disease [9–12].

Origins

M. tuberculosis belongs to the Mycobacteria, a group of over 170 species of bacteria most of which live in soil and water. Left to themselves they are harmless, contentedly eating decaying animal and plant material. Only a few species have evolved to become full-time parasites attacking either reptiles, fish, animals or humans. The two most well-known are *M. tuberculosis* in humans and *M. bovis* of cattle [13, 14].

For many years it was thought that people contracted TB by drinking the milk of cows. In Neolithic times, about 10,000 years ago, when people began domesticating animals, they could have been infected with the bacterium *M. bovis* from cows. The theory proposed that the bacterium then mutated, evolved and adapted to life in humans, becoming *M. tuberculosis*. In fact, it is unfair to place the blame on cows; it was humans who passed their TB to cows during the domestication process. Genetic studies clearly show that *M. tuberculosis* is a much older strain and that *M. bovis* is descended from it. People can develop a form of TB from unpasteurised milk or milk products of cows infected with *M. bovis*. It causes infection of the gastrointestinal tract and accounts for about 1% of all TB cases [15–17].

The date when TB first became a serious human disease is unclear. One possibility is that it may have caused diseases in our distant ancestors hundreds of thousands of years ago and evolved with us since then. Alternatively, TB may have emerged some 40,000–70,000 years ago, at the time of the great Out-of-Africa human migration. It has also been suggested that TB only began infecting humans between 2000 and 6000 years ago. Whatever the exact timing, human TB has been around for at least several thousand years [18–20].

During its evolution in humans *M. tuberculosis* has lost many of its genes, most likely to evade destruction by the body's natural defence mechanisms. It compensates for this deficit by exploiting human genes that have the same function. This means that it can only survive and multiply within human cells; it is a professional parasite [21].

Method of Transmission

Tuberculosis is mainly spread by the cough of an infected person. This produces aerosols (tiny droplets of fluid) which contain the TB bacterium. The droplets are small enough to drift about in air currents. The risk that an infected person will transmit disease depends on the frequency and the force of coughing, the infectiousness of the droplets and the frequency and duration of close contact between infected and susceptible individuals [22–24].

Individuals vary is their susceptibility to TB. On average about 50% of close contacts of diagnosed cases do not become infected. This is largely due to their genes, as some people are naturally resistant to TB. But individual level factors such as HIV infection, smoking, heavy alcohol use, malnutrition and overcrowding also influence the disease risk. Environmental factors are also important, as high humidity, low levels of UV exposure and indoor areas with limited air flow increase the risk of infection. Institutions, particularly prisons but also homelessness shelters, nursing homes and hospitals can experience large TB outbreaks [23, 25–27].

TB follows a seasonal pattern, with more cases diagnosed in the spring and summer. As the bacterium multiplies slowly, it is probable that the winter months are the high-risk time for infection. In the winter people spend more time indoors, so will be more likely to contract the disease from an infected person. Windows are often kept shut during winter, reducing airflow and increasing exposure to aerosols. Finally, the reduced sunshine in winter causes low vitamin D levels, increasing the risk of infection [28].

When breathed in the droplets containing bacteria travel through the lungs to the tiny air sacks called alveoli at the base of the lung. Here they are swallowed up by the host macrophage, cells whose purpose is to destroy foreign objects such as invading bacteria. However, *M. tuberculosis* has developed strategies to neutralise the attack, taking over the cell's metabolism to produce lots of new bacteria. The infected cell then dies, releasing the bacteria to infect other macrophage. Other cells of the immune system, and more macrophages, cluster round to form an aggregate called a granuloma. Initially it was thought that the human host used this structure to control the bacteria, but more recent studies suggest that M. tuberculosis manipulates it to its own advantage [29, 30].

At about 6 weeks after the initial infection, cells of the host immune system damp down the infection, either killing the bacteria or locking them up so successfully they cannot cause further infection. This occurs in about 90% of infected individuals; they do not progress to active disease. However, in a small proportion of individuals, estimates range between 5% and 15%, the outcome is different. The bacteria escape from the initial site at the base of the lung, and carried by infected macrophage, they travel to higher up the lung. Here they continue to multiply, generating a strong host immune response. This causes substantial localised tissue damage which makes the host cough, transmitting the disease to other individuals and completing the life cycle of the TB bacterium [11, 31, 32].

The Global Spread

Out of Africa?

M. tuberculosis has evolved into nine main lineages, L1–L9. As Africa is the only continent in which all the lineages are presents, it may be the continent where human tuberculosis originated. These lineages could have travelled out of Africa with the successive waves of human migration: L1 to India, L2 to East Asia and L4 to Europe. The lineages L1 and

L5–8 are thought to be ancient strains which may have a lower transmission rate and lower virulence. In contrast L2, L3 and L4 are modern strains. Currently, L4 is the most common strain in Africa, the Americas and Europe, whereas in East Asia L1 and L3 predominate. Oceania has three common lineages (L1, L2 and L4), and West Asia has two (L2 and L4). All the regions are host to several strains [33–35].

Expansion in the Neolithic Period

The increase in the size of the human population in the Neolithic period (10000–3000 BCE) is thought to have helped spread TB. Studies of mummies in ancient Egypt show evidence of Pott's disease, a deformation of the spine caused by TB infection. Bones of people in Syria and Jordan from about 8000 BCE contain evidence of the DNA from *M. tuberculosis*. This indicates that tuberculosis was present at that time. Such cases were also found in Germany, Hungary and Italy 5000–4000 BCE and in Egypt around 3000 BCE [36, 37].

The First Pandemic

The first TB pandemic began sometime in the Middle Ages (500–1400 CE), although the date of onset of is unclear. It has been suggested that the frequency of TB infections may have increased in the late Middle Ages. In Europe many skeletons with DNA evidence of TB have been found, particularly in the period 1100–1500 CE. These findings indicate that the disease was common and widespread across Europe. One possible explanation is an increase in the frequency of contact between communities due to the expansion of trade and local markets. Another is the introduction of high-yield dairy cattle into Northern Europe, spreading bovine tuberculosis in their milk. These suggestions are little more than speculation [38–40].

A good indicator of the subsequent trends in deaths from TB are described in the Bills of Mortality for the city of London. These Bills were primarily developed in the 1500s CE to provide an early warning system for outbreaks of the Black Death. In the 1600s the records were expanded to include all individual causes of death. The data were collected, collated into broad groups and published weekly. They show that one disease, phthisis (a term for TB), accounted for about 14% of all deaths between 1631 and 1731. From 1731 the proportion of TB deaths gradually increased to a peak of 27% in 1791. This frequency of deaths was sufficiently serious for the writer and Puritan preacher John Bunyan to describe consumption (TB) as 'the Captain of all these men of death' [2, 41].

The rise in deaths from TB continued in the 1700s. This is often attributed to the Industrial Revolution, an event that is commonly dated from 1760 to 1820 in England. Coal powered steam engines progressively replaced manual labour as a more efficient, and cheaper way of powering machines. At this time the population size grew rapidly, leading to an increased demand for food. When demand exceeded the supply, prices soared and the nutritional status of the population fell. Another factor was the large-scale movement of people from rural communities to large towns and cities. This resulted in overcrowding. These factors combined to increase the risk of TB [42–44].

As the observed increase in TB deaths began earlier than 1760, factors other than steam powered mechanisation must have been involved. Possibly improved methods of farming may have forced agricultural workers to seek employment in cities. An increase in the use of water powered machines could also have increased productivity. Thus, rather than a dramatic transformation, there was probably a sustained trend to the increased mechanisation that culminated in the use of coal to power the machinery. This would also explain why France experience a substantial increase in mortality from TB that preceded their Industrial Revolution by at least 100 years [42, 45, 46].

As the 1700s were a time of the increasingly rapid spread of TB, so the 1800s witnessed its decline. The London Bills of Mortality indicate a rapid fall in the proportion of deaths due to TB from 27% in 1801 to 12% in 1841. For the next 100 years mortality from TB continued to fall in industrialised countries. This was seen most clearly from data for England and Wales: the death rate fell progressively from 300 per 100,000 people in 1850 to 10 per 100,000 in 1960. The United States experienced a similar trend in TB deaths between 1900 and 1960. These decreases were in large part due to the increase in standards of living:

higher wages, better nutrition and reduction in overcrowding. The confinement of TB patients in hospitals, sanitaria or workhouse infirmaries could have reduced disease transmission and contributed fall in mortality rates [41, 47–49].

The Periods of Hope and Neglect

The dramatic reduction in death rates, and two important medical discoveries, generated hope that TB could be controlled. The first advance was the development of a vaccine by two French scientists: Albert Calmette and Camille Guerin. In the early years of the twentieth century they adapted the bacterium that infects cows, *M. bovis*, to produce a strain that could infect humans without causing disease. Trials of the vaccine in the 1920s showed that it was safe and effective. It was named as bacille Calmette-Guerin—BCG—in honour of the two scientists. The vaccine has been in use for over a hundred years, but with mixed results. In some populations it provides up to 80% protection from infection, and in others it has only limited impact. It is least effective in tropical countries [50, 51].

The discovery of antibiotics to treat TB further increased hopes of controlling TB. Streptomycin was shown to be reduce TB mortality in 1944, and a few years later the combination of streptomycin with isoniazid was found to be even more effective. In the 1960s and 1970s, a four-drug cocktail (isoniazid, pyrazinamide, ethambutol and rifampicin) proved to be highly effective. The key to its success was that the drugs have different mechanisms of action, so they work synergistically. This is the standard first-line treatment for TB. The drawback is that the drugs should be taken every day over a period of 6–8 months. The treatment is lengthy because a small number of TB bacteria can survive for extended periods even in the presence of antibiotics. The World Health Organization (WHO) adopted a strategy to ensure maximum benefit from this course of treatment. It focuses on careful case detection, a sustained supply of the drugs and direct observation of treatment to promote compliance. It is referred to as DOTS (the Directly Observed Treatment Strategy) and is recognised as a breakthrough in the control of TB. Although uptake was initially slow, by the year 2000 almost 150 countries were implementing DOTS [52–54].

The advances in prevention and treatment and the continuing fall in mortality rates in many countries in the 1950s led to discussions whether TB could be eradicated globally. Some counselled against this, saying that because infection rates were so high in Africa, Asia and South America there was little prospect of success. Others accepted that mortality rates were high in many regions but proposed that eradication was a worthwhile goal even if it took 100 years. The reality was that by the 1980s high-income countries had lost interest in TB because their mortality rates were low. This led to a reduction in research funding and the closure of leading research centres. The lack of success of the WHO programme on TB led to it being scaled down in the 1980s, with resources transferred to other respiratory infections. TB had become a forgotten problem [53, 55, 56].

The Resurgent Pandemic

The period of neglect only lasted a few years. The United States was the first country to realise that something was wrong. The number of TB cases, which had been falling year on year, levelled out in 1984 and then started to increase. This led to an investigation by the WHO which found that TB cases had also been increasing during the 1980s in Japan and some countries in Africa. It also revealed that the global burden of TB was substantial: an estimated 8 million new infections and 2.9 million deaths occurred in 1990. A key finding was that most, 7.1 million, of these new infections occurred in low- and middle- income countries. Further, in those countries over 80% of cases were in the economically active age group, 15–59 years. This caused hardship when families lost a wage earner. Three main factors were responsible for the resurgence of TB: undernutrition and poverty, HIV/AIDS and drug resistance. They are inextricably linked, with each augmenting the impact of the other two [57, 58].

Undernutrition and Poverty

Undernutrition is the leading cause of susceptibility to TB. The biological mechanism for this is well established: undernutrition compromises the immune system, increasing both the susceptibility to and the severity of the infection. In addition, infection can lead to undernutrition increasing the risk of further infections. Sinha and colleagues quote a saying from Haiti: 'Giving people medicine for tuberculosis and not giving them food is like washing your hands and drying them in the dirt' [59].

Poverty leads to undernutrition and to poor general health, unemployment and impaired ability to grow crops. It can also make it difficult to access healthcare each day to receive treatment. At the national level, unemployment and the accompanying decrease in productivity reduce the ability to fund healthcare at a time when the need for treatment is great. This combination of factors partly explains why TB rates were high in many countries of South-East Asia and Africa [60, 61].

HIV

Coinfection with HIV and TB is common. It has been described as 'an immediate and grave public health and socioeconomic threat'. It led the WHO to declare in 1993 that TB was a global health emergency. The problem is that TB and HIV act synergistically to increase the risk of illness and death. The virus that causes AIDS severely weakens the body's immune response, making it much more susceptible to TB infection. In its turn, the TB bacterium also promotes multiplication of the HIV virus leading more quickly to severe disease and death. Data for 2020 showed that over 200,000 deaths from TB were among people living with HIV. This problem is greatest in Africa, with the highest rates in Lesotho, Zimbabwe, South Africa and Zambia [62–64].

Drug Resistance

Over the last 30 years bacterial resistance to the drugs for treating TB has become a major challenge. As bacteria multiply they mutate and on very rare occasions they become resistant to a drug. But as millions of people have been given the drugs for TB, these rare mutations will often occur. Patients with a resistant strain remain infectious and can spread this strain to other people. The first reported outbreak of drug resistance was in New York in 1993: among 239 patients who had been treated for TB, 44% had bacteria which were resistant to at least one of the four drugs used in first-line treatment. Several factors exacerbate the problem drug resistance: inappropriate prescribing, problems with the supply of the drugs, poor quality drugs, poor adherence to treatment and having had a previous TB infection. By 2019 over half a million patients had a drug-resistant form of TB, although the total had fallen to about 400,000 by 2022. To cope with this problem new anti-tuberculosis drugs have been developed and are used as second-line treatments, but they are costly, require longer treatment periods and are less effective. Research to develop effective drugs which require shorter treatment times is underway but has not yet been successful [65–67].

Current Status

Over the period 2010–2022 the reported number of TB cases increased from 5.8 million to 7.5 million. Over the same period the number of deaths fell from almost 2 million to 1.3 million. The apparent discrepancy between the trends in cases and deaths is most likely due to successful treatment of those recently diagnosed [66].

In 2022 the greatest burden of TB infection fell on South-East Asia. Just over half of the global cases were from six countries in that region. India was dominant with 27% of the total, then Indonesia with 10%. China, the Philippines, Pakistan and Bangladesh also contributed. In Africa two countries, Nigeria and the Democratic Republic of Congo, accounted for 7.5% of global cases [66].

Since it first declared TB as an international health emergency in 1993, WHO has played a major role in highlighting the problem and seeking international commitment to tackle it. These began with the implementation of the Directly Observed Treatment Strategy (DOTS). Then WHO launched a programme to control TB. Initially it was called the Global Plan to Stop TB, but was relaunched as the End TB Strategy in 2014. Taking 2015 as the baseline and 2035 as the completion date, it aimed to reduce the frequency of new cases by 90% and deaths by 95%. A third aim was to ensure that 0% of people with TB suffered catastrophic financial loss due to medical costs or unemployment. Several intermediate dates were also set to monitor progress at 2020, 2025 and 2030. The most recent update in 2024 assessed whether the 2025 targets could be met. It showed that by 2022 the case numbers had fallen by 8% against a planned 50% reduction and deaths reduced by only 19% against the intended 75%. The proportion of people with TB that faced catastrophic costs of treatments was 49%, although the aim was to reduce this to 0%. Even making allowance for the disruption caused by Covid-19, it is clear that the 2025 targets will not be met. Given current progress, it is very unlikely that the 2035 targets will be met either. A possible explanation is shortage of funds. The plan was that $13 billion would be provided annually by 2022, but only $5.8 billion was available. Funding targets of $22 billion annually by 2027 and $35 billion by 2030 appear unattainable [61, 66, 68].

When Will the Pandemic End?

TB was recognised as a serious problem 300 years ago and it remains one today. With increasing prosperity, the frequency of infection fell rapidly in the industrialised countries during the nineteenth and twentieth centuries. Now it is the low- and middle-income countries that suffer from high rates of TB.

The great hope for TB control is that more effective vaccines for prevention, new drugs for treatment and better diagnostic tests will soon become available. To date many promising candidate vaccines have been identified, but none has yet reached the standards required for clinical use. Research is also underway to develop and test new drugs. So far 17 promising drugs are moving towards testing in clinical trials, so there is optimism that new more effective non-toxic drugs will become available in the near future [69–71].

Diagnostic testing is recognised as a 'weak link' in efforts to control the TB pandemic. If the disease is not recognised, it cannot be treated. An estimated 2.9 million people fall into this category each year. The commonly used method is to look at a sputum (spit) sample under a microscope. It is cheaper but very much less sensitive than the new molecular diagnostic tests recommended by the World Health Organization. What is lacking is the political will and the funding to upgrade testing facilities to ensure that all cases of TB are identified [72].

Considerable effort and a great deal of money have been expended on tackling TB, and substantial progress has been made. But there are major hurdles to be overcome. Poverty, undernutrition, HIV and drug resistance are driving the ongoing spread of TB. Overcoming these will be difficult, given the large gap between funding required and that provided. Added to this is the uncertainty of whether current research programmes will deliver effective new vaccines and treatments. As there are currently over 10 million new cases and 1 million deaths from TB each year, it is fair to say that the end of TB is not in sight.

References

1. Lawlor, C., & Suzuki, A. (2000). The disease of the self: Representing consumption, 1700-1830. *Bulletin of the History of Medicine, 74*(3), 458–494.
2. Frith, J. (2014). History of tuberculosis part 1 - phthisis, consumption and the White plague. *Journal of Military and Veterans' Health, 22*, 29–35.
3. Jay, V. (2001). The legacy of Robert Koch. *Archives of Pathology & Laboratory Medicine, 125*(9), 1148–1149.
4. Campbell, I. A., & Bah-Sow, O. (2006). Pulmonary tuberculosis: Diagnosis and treatment. *BMJ, 332*(7551), 1194–1197.
5. Tiemersma, E. W., van der Werf, M. J., Borgdorff, M. W., Williams, B. G., & Nagelkerke, N. J. (2011). Natural history of tuberculosis: duration and

fatality of untreated pulmonary tuberculosis in HIV negative patients: A systematic review. *PLoS One, 6*(4), e17601.
6. Peto, H. M., Pratt, R. H., Harrington, T. A., LoBue, P. A., & Armstrong, L. R. (2009). Epidemiology of extrapulmonary tuberculosis in the United States, 1993-2006. *Clinical Infectious Diseases, 49*(9), 1350–1357.
7. Grzybowski, S., & Allen, E. A. (1995). History and importance of scrofula. *Lancet, 346*(8988), 1472–1474.
8. Kruijshaar, M. E., & Abubakar, I. (2009). Increase in extrapulmonary tuberculosis in England and Wales 1999-2006. *Thorax, 64*(12), 1090–1095.
9. Houben, R. M., & Dodd, P. J. (2016). The global burden of latent tuberculosis infection: A re-estimation using mathematical modelling. *PLoS Medicine, 13*(10), e1002152.
10. Emery, J. C., Richards, A. S., Dale, K. D., McQuaid, C. F., White, R. G., Denholm, J. T., et al. (1943). Self-clearance of mycobacterium tuberculosis infection: Implications for lifetime risk and population at-risk of tuberculosis disease. *Proceedings of the Biological Sciences, 2021*(288), 20201635.
11. Behr, M. A., Kaufmann, E., Duffin, J., Edelstein, P. H., & Ramakrishnan, L. (2021). Latent tuberculosis: Two centuries of confusion. *American Journal of Respiratory and Critical Care Medicine, 204*(2), 142–148.
12. Rahlwes, K. C., Dias, B. R. S., Campos, P. C., Alvarez-Arguedas, S., & Shiloh, M. U. (2023). Pathogenicity and virulence of mycobacterium tuberculosis. *Virulence, 14*(1), 2150449.
13. Bottai, D., Stinear, T. P., Supply, P., & Brosch, R. (2014). Mycobacterial pathogenomics and evolution. *Microbiology Spectrum, 2*(1), 25.
14. Gluckman, S. (1995). Mycobacteria marinum. *Clinics in Dermatology, 13*, 273–276.
15. Hershkovitz, I., Donoghue, H. D., Minnikin, D. E., May, H., Lee, O. Y., Feldman, M., et al. (2015). Tuberculosis origin: The Neolithic scenario. *Tuberculosis (Edinburgh, Scotland), 95*(Suppl 1), S122–S126.
16. Brites, D., & Gagneux, S. (2015). Co-evolution of mycobacterium tuberculosis and homo sapiens. *Immunological Reviews, 264*(1), 6–24.
17. Kock, R., Michel, A. L., Yeboah-Manu, D., Azhar, E. I., Torrelles, J. B., Cadmus, S. I., et al. (2021). Zoonotic tuberculosis - The changing landscape. *International Journal of Infectious Diseases, 113*(Suppl 1), S68–S72.
18. Drancourt, M. (2014). Looking in amoebae as a source of mycobacteria. *Microbial Pathogenesis, 77*, 119–124.
19. Saelens, J. W., Viswanathan, G., & Tobin, D. M. (2019). Mycobacterial evolution intersects with host tolerance. *Frontiers in Immunology, 10*, 528.

20. Sabin, S., Herbig, A., Vågene, Å. J., Ahlström, T., Bozovic, G., Arcini, C., et al. (2020). A seventeenth-century mycobacterium tuberculosis genome supports a neolithic emergence of the mycobacterium tuberculosis complex. *Genome Biology, 21*(1), 201.
21. Gagneux, S. (2018). Ecology and evolution of mycobacterium tuberculosis. *Nature Reviews Microbiology, 16*(4), 202–213.
22. Turner, R. D. (2019). Cough in pulmonary tuberculosis: Existing knowledge and general insights. *Pulmonary Pharmacology & Therapeutics, 55*, 89–94.
23. Mathema, B., Andrews, J. R., Cohen, T., Borgdorff, M. W., Behr, M., Glynn, J. R., et al. (2017). Drivers of tuberculosis transmission. *Journal of Infectious Diseases, 216*(suppl_6), S644–S653.
24. Melsew, Y. A., Gambhir, M., Cheng, A. C., McBryde, E. S., Denholm, J. T., Tay, E. L., et al. (2019). The role of super-spreading events in mycobacterium tuberculosis transmission: Evidence from contact tracing. *BMC Infectious Diseases, 19*(1), 244.
25. Simmons, J. D., Stein, C. M., Seshadri, C., Campo, M., Alter, G., Fortune, S., et al. (2018). Immunological mechanisms of human resistance to persistent MYCOBACTERIUM tuberculosis infection. *Nature Reviews Immunology, 18*(9), 575–589.
26. Abel, L., Fellay, J., Haas, D. W., Schurr, E., Srikrishna, G., Urbanowski, M., et al. (2018). Genetics of human susceptibility to active and latent tuberculosis: Present knowledge and future perspectives. *Lancet Infectious Diseases, 18*(3), e64–e75.
27. Basu, S., Stuckler, D., & McKee, M. (2011). Addressing institutional amplifiers in the dynamics and control of tuberculosis epidemics. *American Journal of Tropical Medicine and Hygiene, 84*(1), 30–37.
28. Fares, A. (2011). Seasonality of tuberculosis. *Journal of Global Infectious Diseases, 3*(1), 46–55.
29. Queval, C. J., Brosch, R., & Simeone, R. (2017). The macrophage: A disputed fortress in the battle against mycobacterium tuberculosis. *Frontiers in Microbiology, 8*, 2284.
30. Ramakrishnan, L. (2012). Revisiting the role of the granuloma in tuberculosis. *Nature Reviews Immunology, 12*(5), 352–366.
31. Boom, W. H., Schaible, U. E., & Achkar, J. M. (2021). The knowns and unknowns of latent mycobacterium tuberculosis infection. *Journal of Clinical Investigation, 131*(3), e136222.

32. Elkington, P., Polak, M. E., Reichmann, M. T., & Leslie, A. (2022). Understanding the tuberculosis granuloma: The matrix revolutions. *Trends in Molecular Medicine's, 28*(2), 143–154.
33. Ngabonziza, J. C. S., Loiseau, C., Marceau, M., Jouet, A., Menardo, F., Tzfadia, O., et al. (2020). A sister lineage of the mycobacterium tuberculosis complex discovered in the African great lakes region. *Nature Communications, 11*(1), 2917.
34. McHenry, M. L., Wampande, E. M., Joloba, M. L., Malone, L. L., Mayanja-Kizza, H., Bush, W. S., et al. (2021). Interaction between M. tuberculosis lineage and human genetic variants reveals novel pathway associations with severity of TB. *Pathogens, 10*(11), 1487.
35. Wiens, K. E., Woyczynski, L. P., Ledesma, J. R., Ross, J. M., Zenteno-Cuevas, R., Goodridge, A., et al. (2018). Global variation in bacterial strains that cause tuberculosis disease: A systematic review and meta-analysis. *BMC Medicine, 16*(1), 196.
36. Bourke, J. (1971). The palaeopathology of the vertebral column in ancient Egypt and Nubia. *Medical History, 15*(4), 363–375.
37. Buzic, I., & Giuffra, V. (2020). The paleopathological evidence on the origins of human tuberculosis: a review. *Journal of Preventive Medicine and Hygiene, 61*(1), E3–E8.
38. Roberts, C. A. (2015). Old world tuberculosis: Evidence from human remains with a review of current research and future prospects. *Tuberculosis (Edinburgh, Scotland), 95*(Suppl 1), S117–S121.
39. Fletcher, H. A., Donoghue, H. D., Holton, J., Pap, I., & Spigelman, M. (2003). Widespread occurrence of mycobacterium tuberculosis DNA from 18th-19th century Hungarians. *American Journal of Biological Anthropology, 120*(2), 144–152.
40. Manchester, K. (1984). Tuberculosis and leprosy in antiquity: An interpretation. *Medical History, 28*(2), 162–173.
41. Brownlee, J. (1916). Certain considerations regarding the epidemiology of phthisis pulmonalis. *Public Health, 29*, 130–145.
42. The, C. R. (1982). Industrial revolution: A misnomer. *The History Teacher, 15*, 377–384.
43. Komlos, J. (1990). Nutrition, population growth, and the industrial revolution in England. *Social Science History, 14*, 69–91.
44. Lienhardt, C. (2001). From exposure to disease: The role of environmental factors in susceptibility to and development of tuberculosis. *Epidemiologic Reviews, 23*(2), 288–301.

45. Haupert, M. (2019). A brief history of cliometrics and the evolving view of the industrial revolution. *European Journal of the History of Economic Thought, 26*, 738–774.
46. Dutour, O., Colombo, A., & Coqueugniot, H. (2021). Was the rise of TB contemporaneous with the industrial revolution? Epidemiological evolution of TB in France (17th-20th centuries) inferred from osteoarchaeological and historical archives. *International Journal of Paleopathology, 34*, 130–133.
47. McKeown, T., & Record, R. (1962). Reasons for the decline of mortality in England and Wales during the nineteenth century. *Population Studies, 16*, 94–122.
48. Barnes, R. F., Moore, M. L., Garfein, R. S., Brodine, S., Strathdee, S. A., & Rodwell, T. C. (2011). Trends in mortality of tuberculosis patients in the United States: the long-term perspective. *Annals of Epidemiology, 21*(10), 791–795.
49. Fairchild, A. L., & Oppenheimer, G. M. (1998). Public health nihilism vs pragmatism: history, politics, and the control of tuberculosis. *American Journal of Public Health, 88*(7), 1105–1117.
50. Sakula, A. (1983). BCG: Who were Calmette and Guérin? *Thorax, 38*(11), 806–812.
51. Fine, P. E. (1995). Variation in protection by BCG: Implications of and for heterologous immunity. *Lancet, 346*(8986), 1339–1345.
52. Anonymous. (1955). VARIOUS combinations of isoniazid with streptomycin or with P.A.S. in the treatment of pulmonary tuberculosis; seventh report to the Medical Research Council by their tuberculosis chemotherapy trials committee. *British Medical Journal, 1*(4911), 435–445.
53. Raviglione, M. C., & Pio, A. (2002). Evolution of WHO policies for tuberculosis control, 1948-2001. *Lancet, 359*(9308), 775–780.
54. Vasava, M. S., Bhoi, M. N., Rathwa, S. K., Borad, M. A., Nair, S. G., & Patel, H. D. (2017). Drug development against tuberculosis: Past, present and future. *The Indian Journal of Tuberculosis, 64*(4), 252–275.
55. Zaki, M. H. (1971). On the epidemiology of tuberculosis in some selected countries. Highlights and prospects for control and eradication. II. *American Journal of Public Health, 61*(4), 843–854.
56. Myers, J. A. (1963). Can tuberculosis be eradicated? *Chest, 43*, 327–329.
57. Lienhardt, C., Glaziou, P., Uplekar, M., Lönnroth, K., Getahun, H., & Raviglione, M. (2012). Global tuberculosis control: Lessons learnt and future prospects. *Nature Reviews Microbiology, 10*(6), 407–416.

58. Kochi, A. (1991). The global tuberculosis situation and the new control strategy of the World Health Organization. *Tubercle, 72*(1), 1–6.
59. Sinha, P., Lönnroth, K., Bhargava, A., Heysell, S. K., Sarkar, S., Salgame, P., et al. (2021). Food for thought: Addressing undernutrition to end tuberculosis. *Lancet Infectious Diseases, 21*(10), e318–e325.
60. Grange, J., & Zumla, A. (1999). Tuberculosis and the poverty-disease cycle. *Journal of the Royal Society of Medicine, 92*(3), 105–107.
61. World Health Organization. (2020). *Global tuberculosis report 2020*. World Health Organization.
62. Narain, J. P., Raviglione, M. C., & Kochi, A. (1992). HIV-associated tuberculosis in developing countries: Epidemiology and strategies for prevention. *Tubercle and Lung Disease, 73*(6), 311–321.
63. Bell, L. C. K., & Noursadeghi, M. (2018). Pathogenesis of HIV-1 and mycobacterium tuberculosis co-infection. *Nature Reviews Microbiology, 16*(2), 80–90.
64. World Health Organization. (2021). *Global tuberculosis report 2021*. World Health Organization.
65. Frieden, T. R., Sterling, T., Pablos-Mendez, A., Kilburn, J. O., Cauthen, G. M., & Dooley, S. W. (1993). The emergence of drug-resistant tuberculosis in new York City. *New England Journal of Medicine, 328*(8), 521–526.
66. World Health Organization. (2024). *Global tuberculosis report 2023*. World Health Organization.
67. Allué-Guardia, A., García, J. I., & Torrelles, J. B. (2021). Evolution of drug-resistant mycobacterium tuberculosis strains and their adaptation to the human lung environment. *Frontiers in Microbiology, 12*, 612675.
68. Chakaya, J., Khan, M., Ntoumi, F., Aklillu, E., Fatima, R., Mwaba, P., et al. (2021). Global tuberculosis report 2020 - reflections on the global TB burden, treatment and prevention efforts. *International Journal of Infectious Diseases, 113*(Suppl 1), S7–S12.
69. Martin, C., Aguilo, N., Marinova, D., & al e. (2020). Review update on TB vaccine pipeline. *Applied Sciences, 10*, 2632.
70. da Costa, C., Benn, C. S., Nyirenda, T., Mpabalwani, E., Grewal, H. M. S., Ahmed, R., et al. (2024). Perspectives on development and advancement of new tuberculosis vaccines. *International Journal of Infectious Diseases, 141s*, 106987.

71. Fernandes, G. F. S., Thompson, A. M., Castagnolo, D., Denny, W. A., & Dos Santos, J. L. (2022). Tuberculosis drug discovery: Challenges and new horizons. *Journal of Medicinal Chemistry, 65*(11), 7489–7531.
72. Pai, M., Dewan, P. K., & Swaminathan, S. (2023). Transforming tuberculosis diagnosis. *Nature Microbiology, 8*(5), 756–759.

Influenza

Influenza (flu) is a disease that affects people of all ages and in all regions of the world. The common symptoms of flu include a runny nose, fever, aches, chills, headache, cough and feelings of fatigue and weakness. The disease often comes on quickly. Although the symptoms are similar to the common cold, they are often much worse with flu. Some patients suffer greatly, describing the symptoms as 'agony', like being 'hit by a freight train' and even 'I felt I was going to die'. In most people a case of flu lasts for 3–5 days, although a cough, tiredness and feeling unwell may last for up to 2 weeks [1, 2].

The annual winter flu outbreaks usually affect large numbers of people, and many die from it. On average, about one billion people are infected, some 3–5 million become severely ill and 300–500,000 die each year. Most of the serious cases of flu occur among individuals who were obese or had prior respiratory disease. Secondary infection with staphylococcal or haemophilus bacteria is probably the most serious complication of flu infection [3–5].

In addition to these seasonal outbreaks, four major flu pandemics have caused widespread illness and death over the past 100 years: the 1918 Spanish flu, 1957 Asian flu, 1968 Hong Kong flu and the 2009 swine flu.

© The Author(s), under exclusive license to Springer Nature Singapore Pte Ltd. 2025

I. K Crombie, *Major Pandemics*, https://doi.org/10.1007/978-981-95-2081-7_11

Five further outbreaks in 1902, 1929, 1947, 1976 and 1977 have resulted in large amounts of illness, but did not have the global spread or the fatal consequences of true flu pandemics [6–8].

What's in a Name

Illnesses which resemble influenza have been given a variety of names. These could refer to outbreaks of illness in specific countries, for example the Hungarian sickness or the Gallic malady, or to regions of a country such as the Picardy sweat. In France, flu was commonly called *la grippe* (from the verb grippe, to seize) or *la general.* Germany used the term *Blitz-katarrh* (lightning-cold) to describe flu, although they also blamed the English using the term *sudor Anglicus* (the English sweat). More poetic are the descriptions used by Londoners such as the *knock me down fever* and the *punch between the shoulders* [9–11].

The term 'influenza' may date from the Middle Ages, a time when some disease outbreaks were thought to be caused by unusual alignments of the planets and the stars. Influenza derives from the Latin *influentia*, meaning to flow into, indicating that a malign influence spread from the stars to cause illness. Another, more prosaic, suggestion is that it comes from the Italian *influenza di freddo*, the influence of the cold [9, 12, 13].

The Process of Infection

Flu does flow into humans, but mainly from the virus-laden breaths, coughs and sneezes of people suffering from the disease. When the contaminated air is inhaled, the virus infects the cells lining the respiratory tract. Most transmission of flu occurs when close to the infected person. This suggested that the virus was mainly transmitted by large flu-containing droplets, because they quickly fall to the floor once exhaled. But there is substantial evidence that the tiny droplets in aerosols also play an important, if not the dominant, role in disease transmission. They contain more virus than large droplets and they remain suspended in the air for longer. Being close to the infected person is important because aerosols are most concentrated in that space. With increasing distance from the patient the aerosols become diluted reducing the risk of infection. Flu is occasionally transmitted by holding the hand of an infected person or touching a surface on which droplets had fallen. Infection then occurs when the newly contaminated hand touches the mouth or nose [12, 14, 15].

The risk of transmission varies with some characteristics of the infected person. Flu is more likely to be passed on by children and by those reporting more severe symptoms. In addition, a small proportion of new infections come from people with no symptoms. Up to 50% of people with laboratory confirmed infection are asymptomatic, but most of them do not infect other people [16, 17].

Origin and Spread of Pandemics

Flu is caused by a small RNA virus. Three kinds of flu virus can infect humans: types A, B and C. The first two have similar initial symptoms, although type A causes more serious disease and more deaths. Most people have been exposed to type C in early life (they have antibodies against it), but few become ill. There is a fourth one, type D, that so far only causes illness in animals [2, 18].

Human flu pandemics have their origins in the vast reservoirs of type A flu viruses that reside in aquatic birds such as ducks, geese, gulls and terns. As many as 20% of these migratory birds can carry the infection. They usually experience mild disease, although some viral strains can cause serious illness and death. The virus replicates in the lungs and the intestinal tract of birds and is excreted in high concentrations in their faeces. Other birds then become infected by ingesting surface water contaminated with the material that has been excreted [19–21].

Migratory birds can spread flu viruses over wide areas. They use established routes known as flyways to travel south from northern breeding grounds to avoid the harsh winters. There are many such flyways: for example the Black Sea/Mediterranean, the North American, the East Asian-Australasian and the East Atlantic flyways. All have helped spread virulent flu viruses [22–24].

Wild and domesticated birds frequently share flu viruses. Humans acquire the infection by handling live or dead birds, particularly through contact with their faeces or urine. The virus has to undergo several genetic alterations before it can infect people. These enable it to bind to human cells, enter the cells to replicate and then find a way of leaving one human so it can infect another one. The virus also needs to be able to cope with a human body temperature that is 3–4 °C cooler than birds and with the less acidic tissue environment of humans. These barriers explain why successful transfer between birds and humans is difficult; it requires large numbers of close encounters. However, transfer from birds to pigs is easier because they have similar cell receptors. As pigs are more closely related to humans, they can act as intermediaries for the transmission of flu from birds [20, 25, 26].

Pandemics and Immunity

People who survive a flu infection are resistant to further attack from the same strain. Their immune systems would quickly mop up the invading virus. Two viral proteins—haemagglutinin (HA) and neuraminidase (NA)—play the central role in both immunity and in several stages of the infection process. HA attaches the virus to the surface of cells, enabling it to enter the cell. NA facilitates the process of cell entry and also ensures the release of newly formed virus particles that have been manufactured in the cell. These proteins are on the surface of the virus, making them the prime targets for the body's immune response [19, 27].

There are many subtypes of HA and of NA, and these are given numerical subscripts such as H1, H2 and N1, N2. So far 16 different types of HA, numbered H1 to H16, have been identified in aquatic birds (there are another two HA subtypes, but these are found only in bats). Similarly there are nine types of NA, numbered N1 to N9, that infect birds (plus another two also in bats) [6].

Pandemics begin when novel combinations of the HA and NA proteins infect humans. (Each subtype of HA and NA is sufficiently distinct that immunity against one subtype provides no protection against being infected by a different one.) Examples of previous combinations that have successfully spread to humans are H1N1, H3N2 and H2N2. The process of swopping different HA and NA subtypes is possible because of two features of flu viruses. First, their genetic material, RNA, is organised in eight separate segments, with the HA and NA proteins each having their own segment. Second, when a cell is simultaneously infected by two different subtypes of virus, the segments can be swapped. The technical term for this is reassortment. A new virus can be formed by the mixing segments of flu strains from different animals. There are several new strains of flu that have been created by reassortment events between viruses of birds and pigs, birds and humans or pigs and humans. There are even instances of triple reassortment involving bird, pig and human viruses. The trouble with reassortment is that it can create a virus with new combinations of the HA and NA subtypes to which human have no immunity. These can be the source of new pandemics [28].

Major Outbreaks and Pandemics before the Twentieth Century

Historical records from about 400 BCE to 1500 CE describe several large outbreaks of disease that might have been influenza. There is more certainty about an outbreak that began in Asia in 1580 and subsequently spread across Europe and into North America. After that there were roughly three or four large outbreaks of flu every 100 years. Two of them were large enough to deserve the term 'pandemic'. One began in China in 1830 and spread through Southeast Asia and to Russia, Europe and North America. The other, in 1889, appears to have begun in Russia and then made its way across Europe and into North America, killing about one million people. But neither of these outbreaks was not as destructive as the 1918–1920 pandemic [29, 30].

The 1918–1920 Spanish Flu

The Spanish flu of 1918–1920 ranks among the deadliest pandemics in human history. Estimates of the number who died from flu range from 17 million to 100 million. This pandemic stands out as being the most infectious and virulent form of all flu pandemics. To be fair to it, the virus was not the sole cause of death; secondary infection with bacterial pneumonia, mainly *Streptococcus pneumoniae*, could have contributed to as many as 95% of the deaths [31–33].

Perhaps surprisingly, the Spanish flu did not originate in Spain. During the First World War, many countries had strict censorship and did not report on deaths from flu. Spain, as a non-combatant, had a free press and its newspapers reported the progress of the pandemic. The disease was then wrongly associated with Spain. Although the label Spanish flu is incorrect, it is so common in popular and scientific literature that it will be used here [34].

The pandemic spread round the world in three waves. The first wave, which started in the northern hemisphere in spring 1918, was comparatively mild. Most of the deaths occurred among the elderly. It was quickly followed, in August, by the second and most devastating wave. This spread around the world in 5 months and mainly killed young adults. The final wave, which started in early 1919, was less severe and affected fewer countries, but also mainly killed young adults [31, 32, 35].

Death was not the only concern. The vast numbers of flu victims overwhelmed healthcare systems, at a time when there were no effective treatments or vaccine. Many unproven remedies were used, such as turpentine, opium, iodine, salt water and Bovril. Drinking carbolic acid was also recommended, but this was quickly abandoned because it was poisonous. Some so-called vaccines were produced, but these were ineffective. As the virus that causes flu had not been identified at that time, it was not possible to develop a vaccine to prevent infection [36–38].

Origin

The origin of the 1918 Spanish flu pandemic is unclear. A human adapted flu virus may have acquired a novel H1 segment from aquatic birds some time before 1907. Then, in a reassortment event in 1916, it acquired the avian N1 segment together with some other genes. Alternatively, a virus could have circulated in pigs for several years and crossed to humans shortly before 1918. Then again, it may have been transferred directly from birds just before the pandemic began. The only certainty is that a virulent H1N1 virus emerged sometime before the spring of 1918 [20, 39, 40].

Three possible locations have been suggested for the geographical source of the pandemic: the United States, Europe and China. New York may have experienced a warning wave of influenza in the winter of 1917–1918. This was followed by an outbreak among army recruits at Camp Funston, Kansas, on 5 March 1918. From there it could have spread through army training centres and then been carried to France in American troop ships, to be spread across Europe by June 2018 [34, 40, 41].

Europe, specifically northern France, is a strong contender as the source of the pandemic. During the winter of 1916/17, British troops stationed in Etaples on the English Channel experienced an epidemic of what could have been influenza. This was followed by an outbreak of a similar disease at a military camp in Aldershot, England, in the early months of 1917. In both locations the mortality rates were high. Further, many of those who died had a characteristic bluish tinge to the skin of their extremities (heliotrope cyanosis) caused by lack of oxygen. This was a prominent feature of the 1918 pandemic [41–44].

The case for China as the source of the pandemic has garnered limited support. There is evidence of an outbreak in November 1917 of a respiratory disease in northern China. It is thought to have been carried to China by travellers from Mongolia. The disease could have been spread to Europe by members of the Chinese Labour Corps. This was a group of 140,000 men recruited from China in 1916–1918 to support the French and British armies in non-combatant roles. They were needed to replace soldiers who were wounded or killed. Their role was to help dig trenches, build roads, fill shell holes and to move cargo and munitions from ships and trains. Some of these men could have carried the disease to France [43, 45].

The common feature of the three proposed origins is the central role that troops played in spreading the disease. Training camps were seriously overcrowded, as were the trains and troopships that carried them to the war. The battlefield trenches in which they subsequently lived were squalid as well as crowded, ideal conditions for spreading the disease. Troops returning home at the end of hostilities would have carried the disease with them. The First World War played the major role in the spread of the Spanish flu [36, 46, 47].

Three More Pandemics

Asian Flu: 1957–1958

Almost 40 years after the onset of the Spanish flu, the 1957–1958 Asian flu pandemic emerged in the Yunnan Province of China in February 1957. It spread to Hong Kong in April and then to Singapore. Ocean-going ships carried the infection to Japan, India and Australia in May. By June it had travelled across the Pacific to the United States and had arrived in Europe in the summer of 1957. The infection also travelled overland through Asia and the Middle East arriving in Europe at much the same time as the sea-borne virus. Air travel contributed little to the spread of this pandemic. Overall, it took the virus 6 months to circle the world. Although the mortality rate was low, at 0.67%, it caused an estimated 1–2 million deaths. If these estimates are correct, they imply that about 150–300 million people were infected by the virus. This was a highly infectious disease [30, 48, 49].

The Asian flu virus resulted from the multiple reassortment events of an avian flu virus, H2 N2, with the human virus H1N1. By acquiring the avian HA and NA segments, it became a novel human H2N2 virus. It retained most of the other RNA segments from the original 1918 H1N1 strain, making it a partial descendent of that virus. This new subtype of flu mainly attacked people under the age of 65. It is thought that a virus of the H2N2 subtype may have circulated in the late nineteenth century, so those who lived at that time would have acquired immunity to it. About 65 years later, those immune individuals would have retained some immunity to the H2N2 virus when it struck in 1957, hence the low infection rates in older people [30, 50].

Hong Kong Flu: 1968–1970

The next pandemic flu was first recognised in Hong Kong in 1968, only 10 years after the Asian one. It had most likely originated in China a few years earlier, although little is known about the place or time. What is clear is that up to half a million cases had occurred in Hong Kong by the end of July 1968. In August and September the virus travelled across Southeast Asia to Australia, then on to the United States and Europe. Veterans returning from the Vietnam War may have contributed to the spread of the virus in the United States. This virus spread in two main waves, with peaks of mortality occurring in the winter months: December to February in the northern hemisphere and June to August in the southern hemisphere. This was the first flu virus in which air travel helped the spread of infection [30, 51, 52].

This new virus was a subtype H3N2, having swapped the H2 of the Asian flu for an H3 from birds. However, it had also undergone mutations which increased its ability to bind to cells in human lungs. The virus had become much more infectious in its new host but was comparatively mild, causing between 0.5 and 2.0 million deaths. Much of this could be due to immunity to the N2 component of the virus which had been circulating in humans since 1957. There were marked differences in mortality rates across countries of the world. For example, Australia, France and England and Wales suffered higher rates, whereas the United States and Canada experienced low rates. It is not clear why this happened [30, 53].

Swine Flu: 2009–2010

After a wait of 40 years a new flu pandemic began in 2009. The first indication came from reports of hospitalisations and deaths from respiratory disease among young adults in Mexico in March and early April. Between 10 March and 6 April, 591 flu cases were reported in the town of La Gloria in the state of Veracruz. At the end of March two young children in California were hospitalised with respiratory symptoms caused by a previously unknown strain of influenza virus. By 14 April the virus had been identified as a new type of H1N1 [54–56].

This new virus emerged after two complex reassortment events in which pigs played the starring role. These animals provide an ideal environment for generating new strains of flu. They have the cell receptors of both bird and human flu, so viruses from both species can bind to and enter pig cells, enabling many combinations of reassortment events. First a new H3N2 swine flu was created from a triple reassortment of human, swine and avian flu viruses in the mid-1990s. Then sometime before 2009 there was another triple reassortment event. It involved a swine H1N1 strain derived from the original 1918 Spanish flu virus, an avian-like swine flu virus from Europe and a relatively new H3N2 swine flu virus. The result was a novel H1N1 flu virus that probably began spreading in January 2009 [25, 57–59].

This pandemic was initially called the swine flu because of its origins in pigs. But the pork industry objected because that label could harm their business. Their concerns were justified, as many countries conducted mass killings of pigs, or imposed import bans on live pigs and pork products. The World Health Organization then adopted the neutral, but more clumsy, title of influenza A (H1N1). An alternative name was the Mexican flu, but this stigmatised Mexico. The label North American flu was also put forward, possibly to avoid singling out an individual country. In 2015 the World Health Organization put an end to the naming free-for-all by issuing guidelines that discourage the identification of specific people, places, occupations or animals or the use of terms that could incite fear. As the term 'swine flu' was popular in the scientific literature before the WHO guidelines, and continues to be the most common term, it is also used here; with apologies to pigs everywhere [60–62].

This new flu virus spread rapidly around the world. By the end of April, cases had been reported across the United States, in several countries in Europe as well as Israel, China and New Zealand. Recognising the growing threat, the World Health Organization declared a public health emergency of international concern on 25 April. The virus continued to spread so that by 12 May, 30 countries had reported a total of over 5000 cases. 4 weeks later, this had increased to 73 countries and over 28,000 laboratory confirmed cases. This led the World Health Organization to declare on 11 June 2009 that swine flu was 'a full-fledged pandemic' [63, 64].

The pandemic declaration was not solely based on the number of cases; it was also influenced by the speed with which the virus spread round the world. In the previous two pandemics it had taken over 6 months to spread the infection across the globe. Swine flu achieved this in less than 6 weeks. For the first time air travel had become the main conduit for a flu virus. It is easy to see why. Between March and April 2009, over 2 million travellers departed from Mexico to 164 countries [65, 66].

Four months after it began, the disease fizzled out. The concern that a major pandemic was underway was unfounded. On 10 August 2010, the World Health Organization declared the pandemic over. With an estimated death toll of 300,000, it was a major global outbreak, but it caused many fewer deaths than previous flu pandemics. The estimated mortality rates were 1–3% for the 1918 Spanish flu, 0.03% for the 1968 Hong Kong flu and 0.001–0.011% for the 2009 swine flu [67–69].

Inevitably the WHO was criticised for declaring a pandemic that turned out to be a relatively mild disease. One suggestion was that the decision was taken to suit the interests of the pharmaceutical industry. After careful review this view was shown to be unfounded. The other criticisms did raise a key issue: at what point should outbreaks be declared a pandemic? Early reports suggested the death rate from swine flu could be as high as 10%. Later studies found the rates were between 0.25% and 0.4%, still troublingly high mortality rates. Combined with the large number of cases and the rapidity of spread, these early mortality data would create the need for urgent action. The benefit of an early decision is that it enables countries to purchase large supplies of antiviral drugs, to develop and manufacture vaccines and to implement population strategies to reduce the spread of infection. If the disease subsequently faded away, as swine flu did, substantial sums would have been wasted. However, if the virus had been highly virulent, then a delayed announcement would mean vital time to prepare would have been lost. The result would be widespread serious illness and death. As always, it is easy to criticise with hindsight [60, 67, 70].

When Flu Pandemics End

Each of the four flu pandemics of the past 100 years caused disease and death on a global scale for only a few years. Then they gradually became less virulent. For example, during the second wave the Spanish flu killed about 2–4% of those who were infected. By the third wave the fatality rate declined to 1%, and then as the pandemic was ending it fell to 0.1%. The most likely explanation for this progressive reduction in mortality is a process called antigenic drift. This describes how mutations gradually change the genes of the virus. (Flu, like most other RNA viruses, has a high mutation rate.) These genetic changes may make the flu virus less virulent. The result is that H1N1 became a seasonal disease which caused large outbreaks of flu in the winter months of every year from 1920 to 1956 [71–73].

The reign of the Spanish flu H1N1 strain as the dominant form of seasonal flu came to an end with the onset of the 1957–1958 pandemic. This H2N2 strain caused moderately high mortality for a couple of years, and then it became the main cause of seasonal flu, displacing N1H1. In its turn H2N2 was replaced by the H3N2 strain that caused the 1968–1970 flu pandemic. The H1N1 swine flu then replaced H3N2 as the main cause of seasonal flu. The supplanted strains do not disappear entirely; they just play minor roles in the winter outbreaks [74–76].

Flu Vaccines

The flu virus was first identified in 1933. By 1942 a vaccine that used inactivated virus was shown to be effective and licensed for use a few years later against seasonal flu. But it was soon discovered that the virus had mutated (antigenic drift), reducing the effectiveness of the vaccine. To overcome this the World Health Organization introduced a system of trying to keep up with a moving target. It used vaccines developed against the strains from 1 year for use in the following year [77].

In the 1960s a new approach to vaccine production used only the HA and NA proteins of the virus. Another innovation was the use of live attenuated (severely weakened) viruses to develop a vaccine. Currently the flu vaccines incorporate the influenza A (the ones that caused pandemics) and influenza B viruses (the purely seasonal ones). Both inactivated and attenuated vaccines are in use. The vaccines are only moderately effective and typically provide about 40–60% protection against flu. For many years researchers have been trying to create a universal vaccine, one that will protect against all strains of the virus. As always there are several promising vaccines, and it is hoped that an effective one will become available in the next few years [77–79].

The Next Flu Pandemic?

Although previous pandemics have faded away, the flu virus presents an ongoing threat of a new pandemic. There is a vast reservoir of these viruses in aquatic birds, and they frequently engage in reassortment events that generate new strains of flu. Added to this is the high mutation rate which can enable the virus to infect many different species, including humans. Among the many candidates for the next flu pandemic is the avian virus H5N1. It emerged in China the late 1990s, since when it has caused thousands of outbreaks in wild and farmed birds. One estimate is that has killed over 500 million poultry. As of 2024, H5N1 has infected more than 800 people. It has also infected several species of mammals such as bears, foxes, seals and farmed mink as well as dairy cows. Samples taken from cows show that the viruses are mutating to become more infectious in mammals. This raises the concern that the virus could adapt to become better at infecting humans [80–82].

There are several other aspiring candidates for a flu pandemic. A relatively recent arrival is H7N9. It may have originated among poultry in China in 2012. The early strain caused mild disease, but by 2017 it had evolved to become highly pathogenic in these birds. Among humans it has caused over 1500 infections. Several other bird flu virus subtypes (H5N2, H5N6, H5N8, H7N9 and H9N2) have been identified as having pandemic potential. So far, all these viruses are very poor at being passed directly from human to human. But given past experience, one of them could mutate to cause a deadly new pandemic. The problem is no one knows which new strain will emerge nor when it will do so [83–85].

References

1. Jutel, A., & Banister, E. (2013). "I was pretty sure I had the 'flu": Qualitative description of confirmed-influenza symptoms. *Social Science & Medicine, 99*, 49–55.
2. Mosnier, A., Caini, S., Daviaud, I., Nauleau, E., Bui, T. T., Debost, E., et al. (2015). Clinical characteristics are similar across type a and B influenza virus infections. *PLoS One, 10*(9), e0136186.
3. Krammer, F., Smith, G. J. D., Fouchier, R. A. M., Peiris, M., Kedzierska, K., Doherty, P. C., et al. (2018). Influenza. *Nature Reviews Disease Primers, 4*(1), 3.
4. Rothberg, M. B., & Haessler, S. D. (2010). Complications of seasonal and pandemic influenza. *Critical Care Medicine, 38*(4 Suppl), e91–e97.
5. Javanian, M., Barary, M., Ghebrehewet, S., Koppolu, V., Vasigala, V., & Ebrahimpour, S. (2021). A brief review of influenza virus infection. *Journal of Medical Virology, 93*(8), 4638–4646.
6. Shao, W., Li, X., Goraya, M. U., Wang, S., & Chen, J. L. (2017). Evolution of influenza a virus by mutation and re-assortment. *International Journal of Molecular Sciences, 18*(8), 1650.
7. Monto, A. S., & Fukuda, K. (2020). Lessons from influenza pandemics of the last 100 years. *Clinical Infectious Diseases, 70*(5), 951–957.
8. Neumann, G., & Kawaoka, Y. (2019). Predicting the next influenza pandemics. *Journal of Infectious Diseases, 219*(Suppl_1), S14–S20.

9. Jack, W. R. (1919). A note on the history of influenza. *Glasgow Medical Journal, 91*(1), 1–24.
10. Townsend, J. F. (1933). History of influenza epidemics. *Annals of Medical History, 5*(6), 533–547.
11. Campbell, E. (1943). The epidemiology of influenza: Illustrated by historical account. *Bulletin of the History of Medicine, 13*(4), 389–403.
12. Brankston, G., Gitterman, L., Hirji, Z., Lemieux, C., & Gardam, M. (2007). Transmission of influenza a in human beings. *The Lancet Infectious Diseases, 7*(4), 257–265.
13. Kaplan, M. M., & Webster, R. G. (1977). The epidemiology of influenza. *Scientific American, 237*(6), 88–106.
14. Klompas, M., Milton, D. K., Rhee, C., Baker, M. A., & Leekha, S. (2021). Current insights into respiratory virus transmission and potential implications for infection control programs: A narrative review. *Annals of Internal Medicine, 174*(12), 1710–1718.
15. Leung, N. H. L. (2021). Transmissibility and transmission of respiratory viruses. *Nature Reviews Microbiology, 19*(8), 528–545.
16. Leung, N. H., Xu, C., Ip, D. K., & Cowling, B. J. (2015). Review article: The fraction of influenza virus infections that are asymptomatic: A systematic review and meta-analysis. *Epidemiology, 26*(6), 862–872.
17. Cohen, C., Kleynhans, J., Moyes, J., McMorrow, M. L., Treurnicht, F. K., Hellferscee, O., et al. (2021). Asymptomatic transmission and high community burden of seasonal influenza in an urban and a rural community in South Africa, 2017-18 (PHIRST): A population cohort study. *The Lancet Global Health, 9*(6), e863–e874.
18. Skelton, R. M., & Huber, V. C. (2022). Comparing influenza virus biology for understanding influenza D virus. *Viruses, 14*(5), 1036.
19. Long, J. S., Mistry, B., Haslam, S. M., & Barclay, W. S. (2019). Host and viral determinants of influenza a virus species specificity. *Nature Reviews Microbiology, 17*(2), 67–81.
20. Wille M, Holmes EC. The ecology and evolution of influenza viruses. Cold Spring Harbor Perspectives in Medicine. 2020;10(7) a038489.
21. Keeler, S. P., Dalton, M. S., Cressler, A. M., Berghaus, R. D., & Stallknecht, D. E. (2014). Abiotic factors affecting the persistence of avian influenza virus in surface waters of waterfowl habitats. *Applied and Environmental Microbiology, 80*(9), 2910–2917.

22. Si, Y., Skidmore, A. K., Wang, T., de Boer, W. F., Debba, P., Toxopeus, A. G., et al. (2009). Spatio-temporal dynamics of global H5N1 outbreaks match bird migration patterns. *Geospatial Health, 4*(1), 65–78.
23. Bi, Y., Chen, J., Zhang, Z., Li, M., Cai, T., Sharshov, K., et al. (2016). Highly pathogenic avian influenza H5N1 clade 2.3.2.1c virus in migratory birds, 2014-2015. *Virologica Sinica, 31*(4), 300–305.
24. Lycett, S. J., Duchatel, F., & Digard, P. (2019). A brief history of bird flu. *Philosophical Transactions of the Royal Society, B: Biological Sciences, 374*(1775), 20180257.
25. Ma, W., Kahn, R. E., & Richt, J. A. (2008). The pig as a mixing vessel for influenza viruses: Human and veterinary implications. *Journal of Molecular and Genetic Medicine, 3*(1), 158–166.
26. Reperant, L. A., Kuiken, T., & Osterhaus, A. D. (2012). Adaptive pathways of zoonotic influenza viruses: From exposure to establishment in humans. *Vaccine, 30*(30), 4419–4434.
27. Du, R., Cui, Q., & Rong, L. (2019). Competitive cooperation of hemagglutinin and neuraminidase during influenza a virus entry. *Viruses, 11*(5), 548.
28. Gong, X., Hu, M., Chen, W., Yang, H., Wang, B., Yue, J., et al. (2021). Reassortment network of influenza a virus. *Frontiers in Microbiology, 12*, 793500.
29. Morens, D. M., & Taubenberger, J. K. (2011). Pandemic influenza: Certain uncertainties. *Reviews in Medical Virology, 21*(5), 262–284.
30. Saunders-Hastings, P. R., & Krewski, D. (2016). Reviewing the history of pandemic influenza: understanding patterns of emergence and transmission. *Pathogens, 5*(4), 66.
31. Spreeuwenberg, P., Kroneman, M., & Paget, J. (2018). Reassessing the global mortality burden of the 1918 influenza pandemic. *American Journal of Epidemiology, 187*(12), 2561–2567.
32. Johnson, N. P., & Mueller, J. (2002). Updating the accounts: Global mortality of the 1918-1920 "Spanish" influenza pandemic. *Bulletin of the History of Medicine, 76*(1), 105–115.
33. McCullers, J. A. (2014). The co-pathogenesis of influenza viruses with bacteria in the lung. *Nature Reviews Microbiology, 12*(4), 252–262.
34. Patterson, K., & Pyle, G. (1991). The geography and mortality of the 1918 influenza pandemic. *Bulletin of the History of Medicine, 65*(1), 4–21.
35. Beveridge, W. I. (1991). The chronicle of influenza epidemics. *History and Philosophy of the Life Sciences, 13*(2), 223–234.

36. Jester, B. J., Uyeki, T. M., Patel, A., Koonin, L., & Jernigan, D. B. (2018). 100 years of medical countermeasures and pandemic influenza preparedness. *American Journal of Public Health, 108*(11), 1469–1472.
37. Jivraj, N., & Butler, A. (2013). The 1918-19 influenza pandemic revisited. *The Journal of the Royal College of Physicians of Edinburgh, 43*(4), 347–352.
38. Schwartz, J. L. (2018). The spanish flu, epidemics, and the turn to biomedical responses. *American Journal of Public Health, 108*(11), 1455–1458.
39. Worobey, M., Han, G. Z., & Rambaut, A. (2014). Genesis and pathogenesis of the 1918 pandemic H1N1 influenza a virus. *Proceedings of the National Academy of Sciences of the United States of America, 111*(22), 8107–8112.
40. Oxford, J. S., & Gill, D. (2018). Unanswered questions about the 1918 influenza pandemic: Origin, pathology, and the virus itself. *Lancet Infectious Diseases, 18*(11), e348–ee54.
41. Oxford, J. S., & Gill, D. (2019). A possible European origin of the Spanish influenza and the first attempts to reduce mortality to combat superinfecting bacteria: An opinion from a virologist and a military historian. *Human Vaccines & Immunotherapeutics, 15*(9), 2009–2012.
42. Oxford, J. S., Lambkin, R., Sefton, A., Daniels, R., Elliot, A., Brown, R., et al. (2005). A hypothesis: The conjunction of soldiers, gas, pigs, ducks, geese and horses in northern France during the great war provided the conditions for the emergence of the "Spanish" influenza pandemic of 1918-1919. *Vaccine, 23*(7), 940–945.
43. Humphries, M. (2013). Paths of infection: The first world war and the origins of the 1918 influenza pandemic. *War in History, 21*(1), 55–81.
44. Oxford, J., Sefton, A., & Ra, J. (1916). Early herald wave outbreaks of influenza in prior to the pandemic of 1918. *International Congress Series, 1219*(2001), 155–161.
45. Calvo, A. (2015). Forgotten voices from the great war: The Chinese labour corps. *Asia-Pacific Journal, 13*(49), 13.
46. Byerly, C. R. (2010). The U.S. military and the influenza pandemic of 1918-1919. *Public Health Reports, 125*(Suppl 3), 82–91.
47. Erkoreka, A. (2009). Origins of the Spanish influenza pandemic (1918-1920) and its relation to the first world war. *Journal of Molecular and Genetic Medicine, 3*(2), 190–194.
48. Potter, C. W. (2001). A history of influenza. *Journal of Applied Microbiology, 91*(4), 572–579.

49. Nickol, M. E., & Kindrachuk, J. (2019). A year of terror and a century of reflection: Perspectives on the great influenza pandemic of 1918-1919. *BMC Infectious Diseases, 19*(1), 117.
50. Taubenberger, J. K., & Kash, J. C. (2010). Influenza virus evolution, host adaptation, and pandemic formation. *Cell Host & Microbe, 7*(6), 440–451.
51. Cockburn, W. C., Delon, P. J., & Ferreira, W. (1969). Origin and progress of the 1968-69 Hong Kong influenza epidemic. *Bulletin of the World Health Organization, 41*(3), 345–348.
52. Viboud, C., Grais, R. F., Lafont, B. A., Miller, M. A., & Simonsen, L. (2005). Multinational impact of the 1968 Hong Kong influenza pandemic: Evidence for a smoldering pandemic. *Journal of Infectious Diseases, 192*(2), 233–248.
53. Van Poucke, S., Doedt, J., Baumann, J., Qiu, Y., Matrosovich, T., Klenk, H. D., et al. (2015). Role of substitutions in the hemagglutinin in the emergence of the 1968 pandemic influenza virus. *Journal of Virology, 89*(23), 12211–12216.
54. Chowell, G., Echevarría-Zuno, S., Viboud, C., Simonsen, L., Tamerius, J., Miller, M. A., et al. (2011). Characterizing the epidemiology of the 2009 influenza a/H1N1 pandemic in Mexico. *PLoS Medicine, 8*(5), e1000436.
55. López-Cervantes, M., Venado, A., Moreno, A., Pacheco-Domínguez, R. L., & Ortega-Pierres, G. (2009). On the spread of the novel influenza a (H1N1) virus in Mexico. *Journal of Infection in Developing Countries, 3*(5), 327–330.
56. Anonymous. (2009). Swine influenza a (H1N1) infection in two children—Southern California, march-April 2009. *Morbidity and Mortality Weekly Report, 58*(15), 400–402.
57. Webby, R. J., Swenson, S. L., Krauss, S. L., Gerrish, P. J., Goyal, S. M., & Webster, R. G. (2000). Evolution of swine H3N2 influenza viruses in the United States. *Journal of Virology, 74*(18), 8243–8251.
58. Mena, I., Nelson, M. I., Quezada-Monroy, F., Dutta, J., Cortes-Fernández, R., Lara-Puente, J. H., et al. (2016). Origins of the 2009 H1N1 influenza pandemic in swine in Mexico. *eLife, 5*, e16777.
59. Smith, G. J., Vijaykrishna, D., Bahl, J., Lycett, S. J., Worobey, M., Pybus, O. G., et al. (2009). Origins and evolutionary genomics of the 2009 swine-origin H1N1 influenza a epidemic. *Nature, 459*(7250), 1122–1125.
60. Kamradt-Scott, A. (2018). What went wrong? The world health organization from swine flu to Ebola. In A. K. KO & A. Spencer (Eds.), *Political mistakes and policy failures in international relations* (pp. 193–215). Palgrave Macmillam.

61. Enserink, M. (2009). Swine flu names evolving faster than swine flu itself. *Science, 324*(5929), 871.
62. Hoppe, T. (2018). "Spanish flu": When infectious disease names blur origins and stigmatize those infected. *American Journal of Public Health, 108*(11), 1462–1464.
63. Fineberg, H. V. (2014). Pandemic preparedness and response—lessons from the H1N1 influenza of 2009. *New England Journal of Medicine, 370*(14), 1335–1342.
64. Anonymous. (2009). New influenza a(H1N1) virus infections: Global surveillance summary, may 2009. *Weekly Epidemiological Record, 84*(20), 173–179.
65. Anonymous. (2009). New influenza A (H1N1) virus: Global epidemiological situation, June 2009. *Weekly Epidemiological Record, 84*(25), 249–257.
66. Khan, K., Arino, J., Hu, W., Raposo, P., Sears, J., Calderon, F., et al. (2009). Spread of a novel influenza a (H1N1) virus via global airline transportation. *New England Journal of Medicine, 361*(2), 212–214.
67. Versluis, E., van Asselt, M., & Kim, J. (2019). The multilevel regulation of complex policy problems: Uncertainty and the swine flu pandemic. *European Policy Analysis, 5*, 80–98.
68. Simonsen, L., Spreeuwenberg, P., Lustig, R., Taylor, R. J., Fleming, D. M., Kroneman, M., et al. (2013). Global mortality estimates for the 2009 influenza pandemic from the GLaMOR project: A modeling study. *PLoS Medicine, 10*(11), e1001558.
69. Dawood, F. S., Iuliano, A. D., Reed, C., Meltzer, M. I., Shay, D. K., Cheng, P. Y., et al. (2012). Estimated global mortality associated with the first 12 months of 2009 pandemic influenza a H1N1 virus circulation: A modelling study. *Lancet Infectious Diseases, 12*(9), 687–695.
70. O'Dowd, A. (2010). Council of Europe condemns "unjustified scare" over swine flu. *BMJ, 340*, c3033.
71. Carrat, F., & Flahault, A. (2007). Influenza vaccine: The challenge of antigenic drift. *Vaccine, 25*(39–40), 6852–6862.
72. Berche, P. (2022). The Spanish flu. *La Presse Médicale, 51*(3), 104127.
73. Simonsen, L. (1999). The global impact of influenza on morbidity and mortality. *Vaccine, 17*(Suppl 1), S3–S10.
74. Hope-Simpson, R. E. (1981). The role of season in the epidemiology of influenza. *Journal of Hygiene, 86*(1), 35–47.
75. Paget, J., Spreeuwenberg, P., Charu, V., Taylor, R. J., Iuliano, A. D., Bresee, J., et al. (2019). Global mortality associated with seasonal influenza

epidemics: New burden estimates and predictors from the GLaMOR project. *International Journal of Global Health, 9*(2), 020421.
76. Yunker, M., Villafuerte, D. A., Fall, A., Norton, J. M., Abdullah, O., Rothman, R. E., et al. (2024). Genomic evolution of influenza during the 2023-2024 season, the johns Hopkins health system. *Journal of Clinical Virology, 174*, 105718.
77. Barberis, I., Myles, P., Ault, S. K., Bragazzi, N. L., & Martini, M. (2016). History and evolution of influenza control through vaccination: From the first monovalent vaccine to universal vaccines. *Journal of Preventive Medicine and Hygiene, 57*(3), E115–E120.
78. Trombetta, C. M., Kistner, O., Montomoli, E., Viviani, S., & Marchi, S. (2022). Influenza viruses and vaccines: The role of vaccine effectiveness studies for evaluation of the benefits of influenza vaccines. *Vaccines (Basel), 10*(5), 714.
79. Deviatkin, A. A., Simonov, R. A., Trutneva, K. A., Maznina, A. A., Khavina, E. M., & Volchkov, P. Y. (2022). Universal flu mRNA vaccine: Promises, prospects, and problems. *Vaccines, 10*(5), 709.
80. Dye, C., & Barclay, W. S. (2024). Should we worry about a growing threat from "bird flu"? *BMJ, 385*, q1199.
81. Leung, K., Lam, T. T. Y., & Wu, J. T. (2023). Controlling avian influenza. *BMJ, 380*, 560.
82. Hou, Y., Deng, G., Cui, P., Zeng, X., Li, B., Wang, D., et al. (2024). Evolution of H7N9 highly pathogenic avian influenza virus in the context of vaccination. *Emerging Microbes & Infections, 13*(1), 2343912.
83. Shi, Z., Wei, L., Wang, P., Wang, S., Liu, Z., Jiang, Y., et al. (2022). Spatiotemporal spread and evolution of influenza a (H7N9) viruses. *Frontiers in Microbiology, 13*, 1002522.
84. Sutton, T. C. (2018). The pandemic threat of emerging H5 and H7 avian influenza viruses. *Viruses, 10*(9), 461.
85. Liu, W. J., Wu, Y., Bi, Y., Shi, W., Wang, D., Shi, Y., et al. (2022). Emerging HxNy Influenza A Viruses. *Cold Spring Harbor Perspectives in Medicine, 12*(2), a038406.

HIV/AIDS: A Thriving Pandemic

Introduction

In June 1981, a handful of cases of an unusual type of pneumonia signalled the start of what would become a disastrous pandemic. Five young homosexual men in the Los Angeles area were suffering from a pneumonia caused by the bacterium *Pneumocystis carinii.* They also had fungal and viral infections. What no-one knew was that a deadly new virus, HIV (human immunodeficiency virus), was the underlying cause of the pneumonia. Some forty years on, and 88 million people have been infected with the virus and over 42 million people have died from it. Currently about 40 million people are living with HIV, and one of them dies from it every minute. HIV infection is an ongoing catastrophe [1].

The Onset of a Pandemic

The initial cases caused concern because healthy young adults are not normally infected by these bacteria, viruses and fungi. Another worrying sign was that two of them died within 3 months of the pneumonia

© The Author(s), under exclusive license to Springer Nature Singapore Pte Ltd. 2025

I. K Crombie, *Major Pandemics*, https://doi.org/10.1007/978-981-95-2081-7_12

diagnosis. Further investigation showed that the men did not know each other, although all reported using inhaled drugs. The study concluded that some exposure was weakening the immune response, increasing susceptibility to infection [2].

A month later 26 cases of a rare form of cancer, Kaposi's sarcoma, were identified in young homosexual men from New York City and California. In addition, a further ten cases of the unusual pneumonia had been identified in young homosexual men. What made these findings more surprising is that both *Pneumocystis carinii* and Kaposi's sarcoma usually occur in older men. Again, suppression of the immune system was thought to increase susceptibility to these diseases [3].

By December 1981 more than 160 cases with *Pneumocystis carinii* or Kaposi's sarcoma had been identified, with five or six new cases occurring each week. They were almost all young homosexual men, although there was one woman. Most lived in large cities and reported using drugs. Over one third of the cases had died. A review revealed that a variety of bacteria, viruses and fungi were infecting the young men and concluded that 'the normal defenses are severely compromised'. The immune system has two main components which protect against infection. One uses antibodies which are produced by a type of white blood cell (lymphocyte) called a B-cell. The other uses another type of lymphocyte, the T-cell, which destroys invading microorganisms. It was the second component, the T-cell, which was being attacked. One suggestion was that a transmissible agent, such as a virus, could be responsible for the weakened immune system [4, 5].

The number of cases continued to increase, doubling every 6 months, reaching 593 by September 1982. Analysis of the survival times showed that just over 60% of those diagnosed more than a year ago had died. By 5 years after diagnosis 85% of patients had died. The disease was not limited to the United States; cases were quickly identified in Haiti in the Caribbean and in several African countries in the early 1980s. Western Europe also began reporting cases. By the end of 1987 the disease had been identified in 129 countries across the world [6–8].

Finding the Cause

The rapid spread of this fatal illness made finding the cause a high priority. Much of the early research focused on the lifestyles of homosexual young men, particularly on drug use and sexual activity. The disease was initially given the label GRID, the Gay-Related Immunodeficiency Disease, with the phrase 'gay plague' being widely used. The sudden appearance of this unexplained disease led quickly led to the stigmatisation of homosexual men, with some interpreting it as a punishment from God for sinful behaviour. There were many other theories about the cause AIDS, such as 'a fascist plot to destroy homosexuals', 'a CIA plot to destroy subversives', 'a Soviet plot to destroy capitalists' and 'a capitalist plot to create new markets for pharmaceutical products'. Other popular myths were that AIDS could be contracted from a toilet seat or doorknob, from a swimming pool or a flying insect. But the gay plague and the demonisation of homosexuals were the dominant themes [9–11].

The term GRID was quickly replaced by the more accurate Acquired ImmunoDeficiency Syndrome (AIDS). It was true that in the United States most of the cases (75%) were in homosexual or bisexual men, but many occurred in heterosexual men and women. In addition, most cases of AIDS in the Caribbean island of Haiti were in heterosexual men and women and in individuals with haemophilia. The occurrence of many cases of disease in disparate social groups indicated that the underlying cause was not to be found in the lifestyle of homosexuals. A report in June 1983 concluded that, although the cause was unknown, it was most likely to be an infectious agent that was transmitted person to person by intimate sexual contact. It could also spread through contaminated needles or the clinical use of blood and blood products [12, 13].

The search for the infectious agent that caused AIDS began shortly after the new disease was identified. The main difficulty was that no one knew what to look for. Two groups of scientists who were working independently, one French the other American, guessed that it was, or it might be, a retrovirus. This is a type of RNA virus which can cause cancer in animals. After 3 years of effort, a previously unknown retrovirus was confirmed as the cause of AIDS. It was subsequently named HIV, standing for Human Immunodeficiency Virus. There followed an unseemly argument about who was first to discover the virus. An American scientist insisted it was his group that made the breakthrough. He then patented the virus, which enabled the United States to claim the royalties from sales of a newly developed diagnostic test. The French were naturally upset, claiming that they were first. The dispute was finally resolved by the intervention of French Prime Minister Chirac and US President Reagan, with each group research being recognised as having made important contributions to the discovery of HIV. However, when it came to the award of the Nobel Prize for this achievement only two French scientists, Françoise Barré-Sinoussi and Luc Montagnier, were honoured. They were judged to have played the major role in identifying HIV [14–16].

The Process of Infection

The HIV virus can enter the human body by several routes, with each one carrying a different risk of causing AIDS. Blood transfusions carry the highest risk, with 9250 cases per 10,000 people exposed. Mother-to-child transmission during pregnancy and childbirth is also very high risk (2260 per 10,000). Needle sharing during injecting drug use carries moderate to high to risk (63 per 10,000) [17].

The risk from sexual intercourse differs for anal (higher) compared to vaginal intercourse (lower) as the lining of the rectum (anal intercourse) is thinner and less well lubricated than the vagina. This makes it more likely that small tears could occur and allow the virus to enter the bloodstream. The risk also depends on whether the person inserting the penis has HIV or whether the one receiving it is infected. Thus, anal intercourse has a high risk (138 per 10,000) if the person who inserts the penis has HIV. The risk is much lower (11 per 10,000) if the person who receives it has HIV. For vaginal sex the chances of being infected are much less, at 8 per 10,000 for the receptive person and 4 per 10,000 for the insertive one. Although the risks of sexual intercourse appear low compared to blood transfusions, this does not mean it causes fewer infections. Sexual intercourse is very much more frequent and is responsible for most of the infections [17].

Replication of the Virus

Once the virus is transmitted to a new person, it invades the mucosal tissue (the lining) of the orifice being used. The virus uses spikes on its surface to bind to specific sites on mucosal cells. It enters the cell by fusing with the outer membrane, and begins the process of replication. The newly produced viruses then invade the cells of the human immune system, particularly the $CD4^+$ T-cells. These cells play an important part in the immune response to infections and their destruction weakens the host's ability to tackle the virus. This makes those with the infection susceptible to a diverse array of bacteria, viruses and fungi [18–20].

The genetic material of HIV is RNA, so to make new virus particles the RNA is first converted into DNA using an enzyme called reverse transcriptase. The DNA version then inserts itself into the host cell DNA. From there the integrated virus hijacks some of the host cell's biochemical processes to make the components of new virus particles. The components are assembled to make new virus particles, which bud out through the host cell membrane. New RNA virus particles can be detected 2 days after the initial infection, although the peak level of virus production does not occur until 3 to 6 weeks later. Each infected cell produces between 400,000 and 2.5 million new viral particles. These new virus particles spread to lymph nodes and then throughout the body [21, 22].

The period of rapid increase in new virus particles coincides with the onset of symptoms of primary HIV-1 infection. These include fever fatigue and muscle pain as well as skin rash and headache. After the initial symptoms there is a long incubation period before the onset of AIDS, although the length of this varies greatly between individuals. About 20% develop AIDS after 2 years, 50% by 8 years and 80% by 12 years. In the absence of treatment about half of those with AIDS die within 2 years and 80% within 6 years [23].

The Origin and the Spread of HIV-1

The emergence and rapid spread of this deadly disease led to an intensive search for the origin of the AIDS virus. The ultimate success of this endeavour is a major achievement of genetic detective work. The first clue emerged in 1984 when a virus similar to HIV was identified in captive rhesus macaque monkeys; they also had symptoms similar to AIDS. Similar viruses were soon found in monkeys and apes from Africa. We now know that are more than 40 types of these viruses. They are referred to as Simian Immunodeficiency Viruses (SIV) [24, 25].

Although each type of SIV usually infects a particular species of monkey or ape, some animals are host to more than one type of SIV. Many instances of cross-species transmission between monkeys and apes have occurred. For example, chimpanzees often hunt monkeys for their meat and can acquire a new SIV in the process. Monkeys and apes with SIV usually have high levels of virus in their bodies, although very few develop AIDS-like symptoms. These animals have coexisted with SIV for millions of years, allowing them to develop mechanisms to protect themselves from the consequences of infection [24, 26].

Humans acquired HIV from bushmeat, the flesh of wild animals caught to be eaten. Bushmeat provides an important source of protein and of income, as hunters can sell the meat. Monkeys and apes are often killed for their meat. As the prevalence of SIV in these animals can be high, in many species up to 80% can be infected, there are many opportunities for SIV to infect humans. However, the virus will seldom thrive in the new host because of the difficulty of adapting to the biochemical environment and the immune system of a different species. To be able to infect a human the virus needs to have acquired several key mutations and to have exchanged bits of RNA with other strains SIV. This combination of events is very unlikely to occur. That is why there have only been four occasions in which the SIV virus has successfully jumped into humans to become HIV-1. This has resulted in four closely related virus strains that have been labelled M, N, O, P [26–28].

Almost all almost all cases of AIDS are caused by Group M. It came from the chimpanzee Pan troglodytes troglodytes in the south of

Cameroon, a country in central Africa. HIV Group O was transmitted from a gorilla to a human in central Cameroon and is largely confined to Cameroon and surrounding countries (west central Africa). It accounts for about 1–2% of human HIV infections. Only 14 cases of group N have been identified so far. Its origin has been traced back to chimpanzees in south-central Cameroon. Group P is the least successful and only two cases have been identified so far. It probably came from a gorilla and is considered to be a dead-end infection [28, 29].

The Early Spread

The earliest known case of HIV-1 group M was identified from a blood sample taken from an adult male in Kinshasa, the capital of the Democratic Republic of Congo, in 1959. At first it was suggested that the HIV-1 pandemic might have begun in this area, but subsequent studies have shown that it most likely originated in southern Cameroon in the early years of the twentieth century [30, 31].

The initial outbreak of group M in southern Cameroon was gradually transmitted between people that lived along the banks of the Congo river to reach Kinshasa, the capital of the Democratic Republic of Congo (DRC). This is where the pandemic really began. The spread of the virus was aided by the actions of the French and Belgium colonisers of West Africa. They created small cities in which there were substantially more men than women. This led to a form of low-risk prostitution in which each woman had a few clients who were visited regularly. In these circumstances HIV infection spread slowly. A well-intentioned policy of giving injections to people with syphilis, sleeping sickness or leprosy also aided disease spread. Needles and syringes were routinely reused, so that blood-borne viruses such as HIV could be passed between patients. To be fair to them, the health authorities were unaware that these viruses existed [32].

HIV Group M also spread to Brazzaville, the capital of the Republic of Congo, and to neighbouring countries in West and Central Africa. Then sometime in the 1950s the virus evolved to become more infectious. It also produced nine subtypes: A to D, and F to K. These subtypes travelled to the rest of the world during the second half of the twentieth century. The pattern of spread is complex with much exchanging of virus strains between countries over several decades. Three main subtypes C, B and A illustrate the different routes by which HIV spread around the world to become a major pandemic [31].

Subtype C is the most common of the subtypes, accounting for 47% of all HIV infections. It has increased in frequency relative to the other subtypes and now predominates in Southern Africa, India and Ethiopia. This subtype may have evolved in the 1950s in a diamond mining region in the south of the Democratic Republic of Congo (DRC). The area has rich mineral resources and attracted migrant workers from the countries of eastern and southern Africa. As migrant workers returned home in the 1970s they spread subtype C to countries such as Botswana, Tanzania and Zimbabwe. This led to an explosive spread of the virus across southern Africa, largely driven by men with multiple sexual partners and female sex workers with their clients. Rapid economic growth, substantial inward migration and poverty also contributed to this health disaster [33–36].

Although it is only responsible for 11% of HIV infections globally, subtype B is most common in Western Europe and North and South America. It started to spread from Kinshasa to neighbouring regions in about 1944 and travelled to Haiti in the Caribbean around 1967. The virus was carried by teachers and civil servants returning home after time spent working in the Congo. From Haiti it spread to the United States in about 1969. Undetected, the number of cases gradually increased until 1981 when HIV/AIDS was finally recognised. In America it was mainly spread by men who had sex with men and to a lesser extent by injecting drug users. But some of those engaging in male-to-male sex also had female partners, so that heterosexual spread gradually increased. The virus travelled from North America to Western Europe and to Central and South America [37, 38].

Subtype A causes 12% of global cases and is dominant in Eastern Europe, Central Asia and East Africa. The former Soviet Union had established strong political links with many African countries and regular exchanges between these regions enabled the virus to spread. It travelled from the Democratic Republic of Congo to Odessa, Ukraine, in 1984 and then to neighbouring countries. The number of cases slowly increased until the collapse of the former Soviet Union in 1991. This caused extensive social dislocation and severe economic decline in the countries across Eastern Europe and Central Asia. The resulting feelings of hopelessness and despair led to a marked increase in substance abuse and prostitution. This drove an HIV epidemic. Most of this was due to a rapid increase among injecting drug users. Subsequently, heterosexual transmission emerged as the main driver of infection in Eastern Europe [39–41].

HIV Deniers

Many individuals and groups have denied that the HIV virus was the cause of AIDS. This movement began in 1987 when Peter Duesberg, a previously respected scientist, claimed that AIDS was not caused by the recently identified virus. Instead, he thought that the virus was merely an innocent passenger. His theory has been repeatedly refuted by experts, but it has gained acceptance among many people. These HIV deniers argue that the scientific findings are simply deep-rooted misguided beliefs. Possibly the most influential of these deniers was Thabo Mbeki, president of South Africa from 1999 to 2008. He argued that HIV was not the cause of AIDS and that medical facts were exaggerated. Further, he claimed that the drugs used to treat disease were toxic and were being promoted to make huge profits for Western pharmaceutical companies. Under his leadership access to these treatments was restricted, even for supplies freely donated. It is estimated that more than 330,000 people died because of lack of access to these drugs [42–44].

HIV-2: Its Origin and Spread

A separate AIDS causing virus, HIV-2, was identified in 1986. It was isolated from two patients from West Africa: one from Guinea-Bissau, a country on Africa's Atlantic coast, and the other from Cape Verdi (500 kilometres off the coast). Both were thought to have contracted the virus by heterosexual contact. The virus was most likely derived from a Simian Immunodeficiency Virus that commonly infects the sooty mangabey monkey in West Africa. Over half of these monkeys in sub-Saharan Africa are infected with this virus. Cross-species transmission of HIV-2 to humans occurred at least nine times, all from the sooty mangabey, to produce groups labelled A to I. The most likely place of origin is the Tai National Park in southwest Ivory Coast. Two of the nine strains, A and B, are responsible for almost all the cases of AIDS caused by HIV-2. Together the other strains account for only a handful of cases [45–48].

Most cases of HIV-2 have occurred in countries in West Africa, particularly in Guinea-Bissau, a country on Africa's Atlantic coast. However, cases have also occurred in a few countries with strong links to this region (e.g. France and Portugal). Compared to HIV-1 it is much less infectious, results in lower levels of virus in patients and takes much longer to cause illness and death. As a result, the risk of contracting HIV-2 is lower than for HIV-1 [46, 48–50].

The Early Global Increases in Cases and Deaths

Diagnosed cases of HIV-1, HIV-2 and their many subtypes increased from five individuals in 1981 to 2.0 million people newly infected in 1990. By 1997 the annual number of new infections had risen to a peak of 3.3 million cases. Annual deaths from HIV followed a similar pattern, rising from a few hundred fatalities in the early 1980s to about 250,000 in 1990. The deaths rose to a peak of 1.8 million in 2004, some 7 years later than the peak for new cases [51–53].

The most dramatic increase was in the number of people who were living with HIV/AIDS. This is the accumulated number of new cases from the start of the pandemic minus the number who have died. It began from a few hundred people in the early 1980s to reach 10 million in 1990 and to about 27 million in 2000. The rapid increases in new cases, deaths and people living with HIV/AIDS galvanised efforts to develop and implementation preventive measures, and to find effective treatments [51–53].

Preventing and Treating HIV/AIDS

Safe sex programmes were launched in many countries from early in the pandemic. As abstinence is an unpopular option, the finding that the consistent use of the male condom can reduce the risk by 80% was important. Promotion of condom use in high-risk groups such as sex workers can increase the uptake of this preventive measure. It is estimated that from 1990 to 2019 condom use has prevented about 117 million cases of HIV [54, 55].

Several other low-cost preventive measures are also effective. Screening blood ensures that supplies contaminated with HIV are not used for transfusions. Treating sexually transmitted diseases of sex workers reduces their risk of HIV infection. As tuberculosis (TB) infection increases the likelihood of contracting HIV, the use of antibiotic treatment to cure TB reduces the risk of contracting AIDS. Awareness raising campaigns, particularly those that involve community led peer education, help increase access to these preventive measures [56–58].

Needle exchange programmes for injecting drug users can reduce the rate of transmission of HIV. Many countries were initially resistant to the use of these schemes. For example, they were banned in 33 US states until 2014. Their view was that needle exchange programmes would 'undercut the credibility of society's message that drug use is illegal and morally wrong'. The state of Indiana was at the forefront of this movement until 2015 when, in the face of a rapid increase in HIV cases, the governor Mike Pence was forced to reverse his previous policy and began funding that needle exchange programmes. In Russia an oppressive drugs policy with restrictions on needle exchange has been responsible for a raging epidemic of HIV. This has spread the infection through the general population [59, 60].

Drug Treatment

By far the most important advance in tackling AIDS is the highly effective drug treatment, antiretroviral therapy (ART). It has transformed HIV infection from a fatal illness to a manageable one. With high adherence to the therapy, the life expectancy of AIDS patients approaches that of the general population. The treatment has to be taken for life because the virus creates a reservoir of infectious particles in a small proportion of CD4+ T lymphocytes. If treatment is suspended, the virus can emerge from these cells and re-establish active disease [52, 61, 62].

ART has two other important benefits. It reduces the amount of virus in the infected person to such an extent that the risk of sexual transmission to uninfected people falls by over 90%. This will greatly reduce the spread of HIV in the wider community. In addition, antiretroviral therapy can be taken by an HIV negative person around the time of high-risk sex. This greatly reduces the chances of contracting HIV even if the partner is positive for the disease and is not taking ART. In men who have sex with men and among heterosexual couples this strategy reduces infection rates by 75%. It has a less effect (49%) in injecting drug users [58, 63, 64].

Tackling the HIV Pandemic

In the early 2000s the global total there was a total of 3.1 million new cases of HIV and 1.8 million deaths. But the burden of HIV was unevenly spread across the major regions of the world. Sub-Saharan Africa was by far the most severely affected. In 2001 it had 2.2 million new cases, 1.4 million deaths and 20.3 million people living with HIV. This amounted to 71% of global new cases, 78% of the deaths and 71% of those living with HIV. Next came South and Southeast Asia with 380,000 new cases, then Eastern Europe and Central Asia with 240,000 new cases. In contrast, Western and Central Europe had 31,000 new cases and North America had 66,000. HIV/AIDS is a global problem, but the burden of disease falls most heavily on low- and middle-income countries. Treatment with ART is expensive, but high-income countries can afford to pay for their HIV positive cases. Low- and middle-income countries, with more cases and less resources, will struggle. Fortunately, two major international efforts have led to reduced costs and to increased funding for HIV treatment and prevention activities [65].

Funding

The widespread use of ART treatment for low- and middle-income countries owes much to the substantial reductions in the price offered by pharmaceutical companies. Those which held the patents on existing drugs granted licenses for generic versions of their drugs to be manufactured and distributed in low- and middle-income countries. Brazil pioneered this approach in 1995–1996, enabling it to provide free treatment for HIV positive cases. The World Trade Association, through the 2006 Doha Declaration, extended the coverage to all low- and middle-income countries. India played the lead role in the manufacture and distribution of these drugs. The impact on cost is dramatic. In the United States in 2020 it cost $38,000 to treat one person for a year, whereas for the generic drugs it is about $75 per person per year. The challenge now is with the newer antiretroviral drugs for which licenses to manufacture the generic versions have yet to be issued [66–68].

Despite reductions in the price of ART, substantial funding was required to implement the prevention and treatment programmes. About 60% of the funding came from the low- and middle-income countries. Much of the rest came from the United States, particularly through the programme which the then US President George W Bush initiated in 2003. The Global Fund to Fight AIDS, Tuberculosis and Malaria also makes a major contribution. The rest comes from other high-income donor countries and global institutions such as the World Bank [52, 69, 70].

As these funding streams came online, the total money available increased from $5 billion in 2000 to $17 billion in 2010. It then rose to an annual $21 billion for the period 2013–2021 before falling to $19.8 billion in 2023. These are colossal sums of money that reflect the severity of the HIV pandemic and the strength of the commitment to tackle it by countries around the around the world.

Setting Targets for HIV/AIDS

Setting specific, measurable and realistic targets is an important tool for improving health outcomes. It helps focus attention on the individual steps to achieve the goal and, with a firm date for completion, it motivates individuals to succeed. The first targets to tackle the HIV pandemic were set by the joint World Health Organization/UNAIDS programme in 2002. Labelled the 3 by 5 campaign, its aim was to treat 3 million HIV cases in low- and middle-income countries with antiretroviral therapy by 2005. The need was great, as less than 5% of the people in Africa and South East Asia had access to ART [71, 72].

This initial 3 by 5 campaign was followed by the 15 by 15 strategy: to treat 15 million people by 2015. It achieved this aim encouraging the setting of the more ambitious 90–90-90 target. The intention was to identify and diagnose 90% of those infected, to treat 90% of these cases sufficiently well so that 90% of those treated would have very low levels of virus. This time the target of 90–90-90 was not quite met by the deadline of 2020. Only 84% of cases knew their HIV status, of whom 87% were being treated and 90% of those were virally suppressed. But it was felt that sufficient progress had been made to justify setting an even more challenging target of 95–95-95 for 2030. This was to diagnose 95% of HIV cases, to treat 95% of them and to suppress the virus to very low levels in 95% of those. If these targets were achieved, then 86% of people with HIV would be virally suppressed, reducing the number of new infections to 200,000 [52, 55, 73].

Impact of the Funding

The preventive measures and drug treatments had a dramatic effect on the numbers of new cases and deaths. From the peak of 3.3 million in 1997 the number of new cases fell to 1.3 million by 2023. The rate of decline was fastest for the decade 2000 to 2009, with a slower fall from 2010 onwards. Similarly, the number of deaths fell markedly from its peak of 1.8 million in 2004 to 630,000 in 2023. Without the intensive efforts at prevention and treatment the improvements would not have been achieved [51–53, 69].

The rates of decrease in new cases and deaths are impressive. But recent data indicate that these falls are not large enough to be able to reach the targets for 2030. An interim aim was to have fewer than 370,000 new cases and 250,000 deaths by 2025. But by 2023 there were 1.3 million cases and 630,000 deaths. The main reason for the limited progress was insufficient funding. To achieve the 2025 targets, annual funding of $29.3 billion was required. Instead, there has been a shortfall of almost $10 billion per year since 2013. Although there have been calls for increased efforts to tackle the global burden of HIV, without a substantial increase in funding it is very unlikely that the 95–95-95 targets for 2030 will be met [52, 69].

Regional Disparities

The global figures conceal marked differences in the trends across the major regions of the world. In sub-Saharan Africa the number of new cases fell from 1.1 million in 2000 to about 450,000 in 2023. Western and Central Africa followed a similar pattern although at a lower level, from just over 500,000 the number of new cases fell steadily to 200,000 in 2023. Asia and the Pacific Islands also had about 500,000 new cases in 2000, and this fell to just over 300,000 in 2023. For the rest of the world the trends varied greatly. The number of cases in Western and Central Europe and North America remained steady at 77,000 from 2000 to 2008, after which the total fell slowly to about 55,000 in 2023. In Latin America the number of new cases was broadly constant at just over 100,000 between 2000 and 2023. But in Eastern Europe and Central Asia the number of new cases increased rapidly from just over 60,000 in 2000 to 120,000 in 2010, after which it slowly increased to 140,000 in 2023. Finally in the Middle East and North Africa the number of new cases remained static at 10,000 from 2000 to 2012, after which it increased to 22,000 by 2023 [52].

The regions also differ in the social groups that have the highest number of new cases. In the Middle East and North Africa most cases are among men who have sex with men, whereas in Latin America it is two groups: men who have sex with men and heterosexuals in the general population. Asia and the Pacific Islands have the same two groups as Latin America. But Eastern Europe and Central Asia have two very different groups, clients of sex workers and people who inject drugs. Western and Central Africa and sub-Saharan Africa both have one dominant group, heterosexuals in the general population. Finally, in Western and Central Europe and North America, men who have sex with men are the dominant group [52].

When Will it End?

Some 20 years ago the HIV/AIDS pandemic seemed unstoppable. Then the massive investment in preventive measures and treatments reversed the upward trend in global cases and deaths. This created optimism that the pandemic could be controlled. From the peak in 2004, the number of deaths each year has been reduced by 69% by 2023 and is estimated that 21 million lives have been saved [52].

The optimism was most clearly expressed in the UNAIDS 2030 strategy which aimed: 'to end AIDS as a public health threat by 2030'. But this only meant that a large reduction in the number of new cases and deaths. Even if the targets are achieved it is recognised that 'the pandemic will be far from over', as there are still many challenges to overcome [52, 74–76].

- The funding shortfall is a major problem.
- Another financial pressure comes from the need to care for the 31 million people currently on HIV retroviral therapy. These individuals will need lifelong treatment and support. Further, people living with HIV are more susceptible to several chronic diseases including diabetes, hypertension, cancer, liver disease, myocardial infarction and mental illness. Their care will be expensive [52, 75, 76].
- Because of barriers to accessing testing and treatment, some 9.2 million people living HIV do not receive antiretroviral therapy. Poverty, stigma and discrimination play a large part in deterring individuals

from accessing care. The result is a large pool of people who could spread the disease [52].

- Tackling HIV among the three high-risk groups, sex workers, men who have sex with men and injecting drug users will be difficult. Many will be reluctant to come forward for testing and treatment. At present there is a shortage of intervention strategies that will assist or encourage them to attend clinics.
- A common bacterial infection, tuberculosis, increases the risk of contracting HIV.
- Finally, HIV is gradually developing resistance to the drugs used for treatment and new therapies are urgently needed [77].

There is broad agreement that a safe and effective vaccine would transform the control of HIV. However, 40 years of active research have failed to provide one. Several candidate vaccines have been tested and found to be ineffective. The reasons for this lie in the biological characteristics of the virus. Not only does it attack the host's immune system, it is also proficient at evading the elements of the immune system that survive. Further, the virus mutates rapidly, creating a constantly moving target for what is essentially a stationary vaccine [74, 78, 79].

It is now recognised that long-term efforts will be needed simply to maintain the progress that has been made to date. Hopefully future success will come from the development of new drugs and an effective vaccine. These could be available 'by the end of the next decade' (i.e. in the 2040s). In the short term, HIV infection will continue to cause illness and death. But if increased funding and the fruits of current research do not materialise, the rate of infection could increase. Whatever happens, efforts to control HIV will need to be sustained for decades to come. This pandemic will not end anytime soon [75].

References

1. UNAIDS. (2024). Global HIV & AIDS statistics — Fact sheet. https://www.unaids.org/en/resources/fact-sheet

2. Anonymous. (1981). Pneumocystis pneumonia—Los Angeles. *MMWR. Morbidity and Mortality Weekly Report, 30*(21), 250–252.
3. Anonymous. (1981). Kaposi's sarcoma and pneumocystis pneumonia among homosexual men—New York City and California. *MMWR. Morbidity and Mortality Weekly Report, 30*(25), 305–308.
4. Durack, D. T. (1981). Opportunistic infections and Kaposi's sarcoma in homosexual men. *The New England Journal of Medicine, 305*(24), 1465–1467.
5. Gottlieb, M. S., Schroff, R., Schanker, H. M., Weisman, J. D., Fan, P. T., Wolf, R. A., et al. (1981). Pneumocystis carinii pneumonia and mucosal candidiasis in previously healthy homosexual men: Evidence of a new acquired cellular immunodeficiency. *The New England Journal of Medicine, 305*(24), 1425–1431.
6. Anonymous. (1982). Update on acquired immune deficiency syndrome (AIDS)—United States. *MMWR. Morbidity and Mortality Weekly Report, 31*(37), 507–508.
7. Rothenberg, R., Woelfel, M., Stoneburner, R., Milberg, J., Parker, R., & Truman, B. (1987). Survival with the acquired immunodeficiency syndrome. *The New England Journal of Medicine, 317*(21), 1297–1302.
8. Piot, P., Plummer, F. A., Mhalu, F. S., Lamboray, J. L., Chin, J., & Mann, J. M. (1988). AIDS: An international perspective. *Science, 239*(4840), 573–579.
9. Fee, E., & Krieger, N. (1993). Understanding AIDS: Historical interpretations and the limits of biomedical individualism. *American Journal of Public Health, 83*(10), 1477–1486.
10. Treichler, P. A. (1987). AIDS, homophobia and biomedical discourse: An epidemic of signification. *Cultural Studies, 1*, 263–305.
11. Heller, J. (2015). Rumors and realities: Making sense of HIV/AIDS conspiracy narratives and contemporary legends. *American Journal of Public Health, 105*(1), e43–e50.
12. Anonymous. (1983). Acquired immunodeficiency syndrome (AIDS) update—United States. *MMWR. Morbidity and Mortality Weekly Report, 32*(24), 309–311.
13. Pape, J. W., Liautaud, B., Thomas, F., Mathurin, J. R., St Amand, M. M., Boncy, M., et al. (1983). Characteristics of the acquired immunodeficiency syndrome (AIDS) in Haiti. *The New England Journal of Medicine, 309*(16), 945–950.

14. Prusiner, S. B. (2002). Historical essay discovering the cause of AIDS. *Science, 298*(5599), 1726.
15. Singer, H. L. (1989). Institut Pasteur v. United States: The AIDS patent dispute, the contract disputes act and the international exchange of scientific data. *American Journal of Law & Medicine, 15*(4), 439–459.
16. Abbott, A., & Brumfiel, G. (2008). Nobel for AIDS virus discovery, finally. *Nature, 455*(7214), 712–713.
17. Patel, P., Borkowf, C. B., Brooks, J. T., Lasry, A., Lansky, A., & Mermin, J. (2014). Estimating per-act HIV transmission risk: A systematic review. *AIDS, 28*(10), 1509–1519.
18. Joag, V. R., McKinnon, L. R., Liu, J., Kidane, S. T., Yudin, M. H., Nyanga, B., et al. (2016). Identification of preferential CD4+ T-cell targets for HIV infection in the cervix. *Mucosal Immunology, 9*(1), 1–12.
19. Shaw, G. M., & Hunter, E. (2012). HIV transmission. *Cold Spring Harbor Perspectives in Medicine, 2*(11), a006965.
20. Engelman, A., & Cherepanov, P. (2012). The structural biology of HIV-1: Mechanistic and therapeutic insights. *Nature Reviews. Microbiology, 10*(4), 279–290.
21. Deeks, S. G., Overbaugh, J., Phillips, A., & Buchbinder, S. (2015). HIV infection. *Nature Reviews. Disease Primers, 1*, 15035.
22. Hutchinson, J. (2001). The biology and evolution of HIV. *Annual Review of Anthropology, 30*, 85–108.
23. Poorolajal, J., Hooshmand, E., Mahjub, H., Esmailnasab, N., & Jenabi, E. (2016). Survival rate of AIDS disease and mortality in HIV-infected patients: A meta-analysis. *Public Health, 139*, 3–12.
24. Peeters, M., D'Arc, M., & Delaporte, E. (2014). Origin and diversity of human retroviruses. *AIDS Reviews, 16*(1), 23–34.
25. Raehtz, K., Pandrea, I., & Apetrei, C. (2016). The well-tempered SIV infection: Pathogenesis of SIV infection in natural hosts in the wild, with emphasis on virus transmission and early events post-infection that may contribute to protection from disease progression. *Infection, Genetics and Evolution, 46*, 308–323.
26. Sauter, D., & Kirchoff, F. (2019). Key viral adaptations preceding the AIDS pandemic. *Cell Host & Microbe, 25*, 27–38.
27. Van Heuverswyn, F., & Peeters, M. (2007). The origins of HIV and implications for the global epidemic. *Current Infectious Disease Reports, 9*(4), 338–346.

28. Hemelaar, J. (2012). The origin and diversity of the HIV-1 pandemic. *Trends in Molecular Medicine, 18*(3), 182–192.
29. Keita, M. B., Hamad, I., & Bittar, F. (2014). Looking in apes as a source of human pathogens. *Microbial Pathogenesis, 77*, 149–154.
30. Zhu, T., Korber, B. T., Nahmias, A. J., Hooper, E., Sharp, P. M., & Ho, D. D. (1998). An African HIV-1 sequence from 1959 and implications for the origin of the epidemic. *Nature, 391*(6667), 594–597.
31. Faria, N. R., Rambaut, A., Suchard, M. A., Baele, G., Bedford, T., Ward, M. J., et al. (2014). HIV epidemiology. The early spread and epidemic ignition of HIV-1 in human populations. *Science, 346*(6205), 56–61.
32. Pépin, J. (2013). The origins of AIDS: From patient zero to ground zero. *Journal of Epidemiology and Community Health, 67*(6), 473–475.
33. Gartner, M. J., Roche, M., Churchill, M. J., Gorry, P. R., & Flynn, J. K. (2020). Understanding the mechanisms driving the spread of subtype C HIV-1. *eBioMedicine, 53*, 102682.
34. Wilkinson, E., Engelbrecht, S., & de Oliveira, T. (2015). History and origin of the HIV-1 subtype C epidemic in South Africa and the greater southern African region. *Scientific Reports, 5*, 16897.
35. Mabaso, M., Makola, L., Naidoo, I., Mlangeni, L. L., Jooste, S., & Simbayi, L. (2019). HIV prevalence in South Africa through gender and racial lenses: Results from the 2012 population-based national household survey. *International Journal for Equity in Health, 18*(1), 167.
36. Hunter, D. J. (1993). AIDS in sub-Saharan Africa: The epidemiology of heterosexual transmission and the prospects for prevention. *Epidemiology, 4*(1), 63–72.
37. Junqueira, D. M., & Almeida, S. E. (2016). HIV-1 subtype B: Traces of a pandemic. *Virology, 495*, 173–184.
38. Gilbert, M. T., Rambaut, A., Wlasiuk, G., Spira, T. J., Pitchenik, A. E., & Worobey, M. (2007). The emergence of HIV/AIDS in the Americas and beyond. *Proceedings of the National Academy of Sciences of the United States of America, 104*(47), 18566–18570.
39. Hamers, F. F., & Downs, A. M. (2003). HIV in central and eastern Europe. *Lancet, 361*(9362), 1035–1044.
40. DeHovitz, J., Uuskula, A., & El-Bassel, N. (2014). The HIV epidemic in Eastern Europe and Central Asia. *Current HIV/AIDS Reports, 11*(2), 168–176.
41. Díez-Fuertes, F., Cabello, M., & Thomson, M. M. (2015). Bayesian phylogeographic analyses clarify the origin of the HIV-1 subtype a variant

circulating in former Soviet Union's countries. *Infection, Genetics and Evolution, 33*, 197–205.
42. Kurth, R. (1990). Does HIV cause AIDS? an updated response to Duesberg's theories. *Intervirology, 31*(6), 301–314.
43. Chigwedere, P., Seage, G. R., Gruskin, S., Lee, T. H., & Essex, M. (2008). Estimating the lost benefits of antiretroviral drug use in South Africa. *Journal of Acquired Immune Deficiency Syndromes, 49*(4), 410–415.
44. Tsikata, P., Pindi, G., & Anaele, A. (2016). The frozen rhetoric of aids denialism and the flourishing claims of a cure: Comparative analysis of Thabo Mbeki and Yahya Jammeh's rhetoric. *South African Journal for Communication Theory and Research, 42*, 378–397.
45. Clavel, F., Guétard, D., Brun-Vézinet, F., Chamaret, S., Rey, M. A., Santos-Ferreira, M. O., et al. (1986). Isolation of a new human retrovirus from west African patients with AIDS. *Science, 233*(4761), 343–346.
46. de Silva, T. I., Cotten, M., & Rowland-Jones, S. L. (2008). HIV-2: the forgotten AIDS virus. *Trends in Microbiology, 16*(12), 588–595.
47. Ayouba, A., Akoua-Koffi, C., Calvignac-Spencer, S., Esteban, A., Locatelli, S., Li, H., et al. (2013). Evidence for continuing cross-species transmission of SIVsmm to humans: characterization of a new HIV-2 lineage in rural Côte D'ivoire. *AIDS, 27*(15), 2488–2491.
48. Visseaux, B., Damond, F., Matheron, S., Descamps, D., & Charpentier, C. (2016). Hiv-2 molecular epidemiology. *Infection, Genetics and Evolution, 46*, 233–240.
49. Azevedo-Pereira, J. M., & Santos-Costa, Q. (2016). HIV interaction with human host: HIV-2 as a model of a less virulent infection. *AIDS Reviews, 18*(1), 44–53.
50. Gottlieb, G. S., Raugi, D. N., & Smith, R. A. (2018). 90-90-90 for HIV-2? Ending the HIV-2 epidemic by enhancing care and clinical management of patients infected with HIV-2. *Lancet HIV, 5*(7), e390–e399.
51. GBD 2015 HIV Collaborators. (2016). Global, regional, and national life expectancy, all-cause mortality, and cause-specific mortality for 249 causes of death, 1980-2015: A systematic analysis for the global burden of disease study 2015. *Lancet, 388*(10053), 1459–1544.
52. UNAIDS. (2024). The urgency of now: AIDS at the crossroads..
53. GBD 2019 HIV Collaborators. (2021). Global, regional, and national sex-specific burden and control of the HIV epidemic, 1990-2019, for 204 countries and territories: The global burden of diseases study 2019. *Lancet HIV, 8*(10), e633–e651.

54. Weller, S., & Davis, K. (2001). Condom effectiveness in reducing heterosexual HIV transmission. *Cochrane Database of Systematic Reviews, 3*, Cd003255.
55. UNAIDS. (2021). *UNAIDS data 2021*. UNAIDS. https://www.unaids.org/sites/default/files/media_asset/JC3032_AIDS_Data_book_2021_En.pdf
56. Marseille, E., Hofmann, P. B., & Kahn, J. G. (2002). HIV prevention before HAART in sub-Saharan Africa. *Lancet, 359*(9320), 1851–1856.
57. Campbell, C., & Mzaidume, Y. (2002). How can HIV be prevented in South Africa? A social perspective. *BMJ, 324*(7331), 229–232.
58. Creese, A., Floyd, K., Alban, A., & Guinness, L. (2002). Cost-effectiveness of HIV/AIDS interventions in Africa: A systematic review of the evidence. *Lancet, 359*(9318), 1635–1643.
59. Weinmeyer, R. (2016). Needle exchange programs' status in US politics. *AMA Journal of Ethics, 18*(3), 252–257.
60. Kalichman, S. C. (2017). Pence, Putin, Mbeki and their HIV/AIDS-related crimes against humanity: Call for social justice and behavioral science advocacy. *AIDS and Behavior, 21*(4), 963–967.
61. Cohen, M. S., Chen, Y. Q., McCauley, M., Gamble, T., Hosseinipour, M. C., Kumarasamy, N., et al. (2016). Antiretroviral therapy for the prevention of HIV-1 transmission. *The New England Journal of Medicine, 375*(9), 830–839.
62. Cohn, L. B., Chomont, N., & Deeks, S. G. (2020). The biology of the HIV-1 latent reservoir and implications for cure strategies. *Cell Host & Microbe, 27*(4), 519–530.
63. Phanuphak, N., & Gulick, R. M. (2020). HIV treatment and prevention 2019: Current standards of care. *Current Opinion in HIV and AIDS, 15*(1), 4–12.
64. Krakower, D. S., Jain, S., & Mayer, K. H. (2015). Antiretrovirals for primary HIV prevention: The current status of pre- and post-exposure prophylaxis. *Current HIV/AIDS Reports, 12*(1), 127–138.
65. UNAIDS. (2010). UNAIDS report on the global AIDS epidemic 2010. https://www.unaids.org/sites/default/files/media_asset/20101123_globalreport_en_1.pdf
66. Waning, B., Diedrichsen, E., & Moon, S. (2010). A lifeline to treatment: The role of Indian generic manufacturers in supplying antiretroviral medicines to developing countries. *Journal of the International AIDS Society, 13*, 35.

67. Hoen, E., Berger, J., Calmy, A., & Moon, S. (2011). Driving a decade of change: HIV/AIDS, patents and access to medicines for all. *Journal of the International AIDS Society, 14*, 15.
68. Heath, K., Levi, J., & Hill, A. (2021). The joint United Nations programme on HIV/AIDS 95-95-95 targets: Worldwide clinical and cost benefits of generic manufacture. *AIDS, 35*(Suppl 2), S197–s203.
69. UNAIDS. (2023). *The path that ends AIDS: 2023 global AIDS update*. UNAIDS. https://thepath.unaids.org/wp-content/themes/unaids2023/assets/files/2023_report.pdf
70. Nachega, J. B., Serwadda, D., Abimiku, A., Sikazwe, I., & Abdool, K. Q. (2023). PEPFAR at 20 - a game-changing impact on HIV in Africa. *New England Journal of Medicine, 389*(1), 1–4.
71. van Herten, L. M., & Gunning-Schepers, L. J. (2000). Targets as a tool in health policy part I: Lessons learned. *Health Policy, 53*(1), 1–11.
72. World Health Organization. (2003). *Treating 3 million by 2005 making it happen*. World Health Organization. https://apps.who.int/iris/bitstream/handle/10665/42845/9241591129.pdf?sequence=1&isAllowed=y
73. UNAIDS. (2014). *90-90-90 an ambitious treatment target to help end the AIDS epidemic*. UNAIDS. https://www.unaids.org/sites/default/files/media_asset/90-90-90_en.pdf
74. Landovitz, R. J., Scott, H., & Deeks, S. G. (2023). Prevention, treatment and cure of HIV infection. *Nature Reviews. Microbiology, 21*(10), 657–670.
75. The Post-2030 HIV Response Working Group. (2024). The HIV response beyond 2030: Preparing for decades of sustained HIV epidemic control in eastern and southern Africa. *Lancet, 404*(10453), 638–641.
76. Althoff, K. N., Stewart, C., Humes, E., Gerace, L., Boyd, C., Gebo, K., et al. (2024). The forecasted prevalence of comorbidities and multimorbidity in people with HIV in the United States through the year 2030: A modeling study. *PLoS Medicine, 21*(1), e1004325.
77. Parums, D. V. (2024). Editorial: Forty years of waiting for prevention and cure of HIV infection - ongoing challenges and hopes for vaccine development and overcoming antiretroviral drug resistance. *Medical Science Monitor, 30*, e944600.

78. Ng'uni, T., Chasara, C., & Ndhlovu, Z. M. (2020). Major scientific hurdles in HIV vaccine development: Historical perspective and future directions. *Frontiers in Immunology, 11*, 590780.
79. Hargrave, A., Mustafa, A. S., Hanif, A., Tunio, J. H., & Hanif, S. N. M. (2021). Current status of HIV-1 vaccines. *Vaccines (Basel), 9*(9), 1026.

Covid-19 and Coronaviruses

Introduction

Covid-19 was an unexpected pandemic. Most countries were unprepared for it, but they shouldn't have been. For several years experts had been predicting that a major pandemic was imminent. Further, in 1969 the World Health Organization introduced the International Health Regulations that required countries develop comprehensive plans to combat large-scale outbreaks of infectious disease. These regulations were strengthened in 2005 (following the SARS epidemic) and again 2016 after a major Ebola outbreak in West Africa. But when Covid-19 struck, 'pandemic preparedness was limited and disjointed, leaving health systems overwhelmed' [1–3].

The consequences of Covid-19 are horrifying. As of August 2024, some 776 million cases and 7 million deaths were reported to the World Health Organization. The United States had most deaths (1.2 million), followed by Brazil (702,000), India (534,000 and Russia (403,000). Many people who became severely ill could not be hospitalised, because the available beds were already filled [4, 5].

© The Author(s), under exclusive license to Springer Nature Singapore Pte Ltd. 2025
I. K Crombie, *Major Pandemics*, https://doi.org/10.1007/978-981-95-2081-7_13

The Early Spread

The beginning of the Covid-19 pandemic was unremarkable. On 26 December Jixian Zhang, a doctor at a hospital in Wuhan city, became concerned about four cases of an unusual form of pneumonia. He acted promptly, notifying the local infectious disease control centre. Two days later a further three cases of pneumonia were admitted to the same hospital. This prompted a systematic search for similar cases. It revealed that the first case had occurred on 16 December 2019, although no one recognised it at the time. By 31 December at least 174 people had been infected. The World Health Organization (WHO) was notified about this outbreak of an atypical pneumonia. A few days later Chinese scientists identified the novel coronavirus that was causing the infection. The Covid-19 pandemic was underway [6–8].

The outbreak in Wuhan city spread across the province of Hubei. But one key event ensured that Covid-19 was quickly dispersed across China. The Spring Festival that celebrates the Chinese New Year begins on 10 January and lasts for 40 days. Hundreds of millions of people travel throughout China to be with their families. Their extensive use of rail and air travel meant that Covid-19 was present in all China's 31 provinces by 30 January [7, 9, 10].

The first case of Covid-19 outside China was diagnosed in Thailand on 13 January. This was quickly followed by reports from other countries which are geographically close to China: South Korea, Taiwan and Japan. By the end of January the infection was prevalent in much of Southeast Asia and North America, Europe and Australia. The number of cases in each country was closely related to the volume of air travel with China. On 30 January 2020 the World Health Organization, which had been carefully monitoring the rise in the number of cases, declared that the Covid-19 outbreak constituted a Public Health Emergency of International Concern. They judged that the rapid spread of the disease posed a serious risk and required an internationally coordinated response [11–13].

By 29 February 79,000 cases were diagnosed in China and 2838 people had died. The infection had also spread to 53 other countries where it caused 6009 cases and 86 deaths. The global cases were unevenly distributed with three countries—South Korea, Italy and Iran—accounting for two-thirds of the total. Less than 2 weeks later the infection had caused 37,000 cases in 113 other countries. The rapid increase in the numbers of cases and in the countries affected led WHO to declare that Covid-19 was a global pandemic on 11 March 2020. By the end of June the number of reported cases was over 10 million, with four countries accounting for almost half of them: the United States (2.5 million), Brazil (1.3 million), Russian Federation (650,000) and India (570,000) [14–16].

A pandemic of this magnitude raises crucial questions about why it spread so quickly, how it caused so much serious illness and death and why is it continuing to cause waves of infection. The answers to these questions lie in the biology of the virus, its remarkable ability to infect humans and almost incidentally cause serious disease. These are properties of the family of viruses to which Covid-19 belongs, Coronaviruses.

Coronaviruses

Coronaviruses are spherical RNA viruses. In an electron microscope they appear as a fuzzy blobs surrounded by spikes. The name corona comes from the Latin term for a crown. It was chosen because the outline of the virus resembles the crown worn by many ancient gods and rulers. The Statue of Liberty in New York Harbour is adorned by the same type of crown. There are many different species of coronavirus, and some have been around for a long time, possibly millions of years. They can infect a wide range of animals, including pigs, horses, cats, dogs, ferrets, rodents, many species of birds and even the beluga whale [17–19].

A key factor in the success of coronaviruses is a molecule on the surface of the virus, the spike protein. It binds to specific receptors on the cell of the host animal, enabling the virus to enter the cell and start making new virus particles. Animals differ in the receptors they provide, so the structure of the spike protein determines which species the virus can infect. This would seem to limit the spread of coronaviruses, but by varying the shape of the spike protein coronaviruses can jump from one species to another. They use two techniques, mutation and recombination (swapping bits of their genetic material, RNA, between viruses) to change the shape of the spike protein. Although almost all of the shape changes will be unproductive, very occasionally one will allow the virus to jump to a new species [20, 21].

Human Coronaviruses

Four coronaviruses have been infecting humans for at least 100 years. These viruses originally came from bats. They cause the symptoms of the common cold and account for about 30% of cases of this disease. But two coronaviruses that jumped into humans more recently cause more serious illness and death: SARS and MERS [19, 22].

SARS

The major epidemic of SARS (severe acute respiratory syndrome) began on 19 November 2002 in Guangdong Province in southern China, and in a few weeks it had spread across south east Asia. The virus probably came from a horseshoe bat, but was passed to humans by a palm civet (a mongoose-like animal). These animals were sold as an exotic food, and most of the early cases were among people who handled, killed or butchered them [23, 24].

SARS caused a flu-like illness that quickly spread across China, and reached Hong Kong, Vietnam and Singapore in February 2003. Within another 2 months it had travelled around the world. The novel coronavirus responsible was quickly identified and named SARS-CoV: with SARS standing for severe acute respiratory syndrome, and CoV is an abbreviation of coronavirus. The SARS outbreak was officially declared over on 5 July 2003. Across the world, 8098 people were diagnosed with SARS, of whom 774 died. Most cases occurred in China (5327) and Hong Kong (1755). Taiwan (346), Canada (251) and Singapore (238) also had many cases. Although short-lived, the SARS epidemic was notable for three reasons. The first is the importance of air travel in the rapid spread of the virus to countries around the world. Then there is the rate at which the disease was spread in healthcare facilities, particularly hospitals. This was due to superspreading, where a small number of SARS cases infect large numbers of people. Superspreading events occurred in Guangzou, Hong Kong, Singapore, Toronto and Beijing. Finally, there is the cost to the global economy, estimated at more than $13 billion [23, 25, 26].

MERS

Ten years after SARS, another new human coronavirus emerged. A 60 year-old man in the Kingdom of Saudi Arabia was hospitalised for pneumonia and subsequently died. A novel coronavirus was quickly identified and serological testing showed that several people in Middle Eastern countries had also been infected. The virus was named MERS-CoV, a Middle East Respiratory Syndrome caused by a coronavirus [27–29].

The most likely source of MERS-CoV is the Egyptian tomb bat. MERS infection is passed from these bats to humans through an intermediate host, the dromedary camels (the single hump variety of camel). Up to 96% of camels in Middle Eastern countries have been infected by this virus. Close contact with dromedaries is the main risk factor for infection, with those involved in rearing, selling camels or processing camel meat at high risk. Consumption of unpasteurised camel milk can also spread the infection. It is thought that there have been hundreds of MERS-CoV spillovers events (camel to human), with only a few resulting in overt disease. A few MERS-CoV cases have led to large outbreaks in hospitals [30–33].

Although MERS can cause severe illness and death, its global impact has been small. As of October 2022, a total of 2600 confirmed MERS cases and 935 deaths had been reported. Some 27 countries have reported cases, with Saudi Arabia accounting for 2193 (84%) of the total. Only five other countries had more than 10 cases: South Korea (186), United Arab Emirates [34], Jordan [28], Qatar [28] and Oman [25]. But unlike SARS, which ended quickly, MERS continues to cause outbreaks because of repeated jumps from camels to humans [35, 36].

The Covid-19 Pandemic

The virus that caused Covid-19 was named SARS CoV-2 because it is closely related to the original SARS-CoV, and it is the second virus of this type to be identified. Common symptoms of SARS CoV-2 infection include fever, a chronic cough, loss of taste or smell, shortness of breath, fatigue and headache [37, 38].

The virus initially invades cells in the lining of the nose and the upper respiratory tract using the spike protein to bind to a specific receptor called ACE2 (angiotensin-converting enzyme 2). It then invades the lower respiratory tract and in some cases attacks cells of other organs. Once inside a cell the virus replicates quickly. The peak of virus production occurs about 5 days after infection, around the time that symptoms begin to appear. People with the disease are most infectious over the period from the day before symptoms start to about a week later [37, 39].

Of those diagnosed with Covid-19 about 80% have mild disease because their immune systems successfully destroy the invading virus. A further 15% have moderate to severe disease in which lung function is seriously impaired, leading to low levels of oxygen in the blood. The remaining 5% have a life-threatening condition called acute respiratory distress syndrome. It is caused by a combination of the damaging effects of the virus and a very overactive and disordered immune response. The system that regulates blood pressure and fluid balance is also compromised. Together these factors cause substantial damage to the lungs and many other organs such as the blood, heart, kidneys, liver and the nervous system. Older people and those with pre-existing medical conditions such as diabetes, cancer and heart disease are more likely to have severe disease. Other factors associated with severe disease include male gender, smoking and obesity [37, 40].

About 50% of people who recover from the infection can suffer from long Covid: enduring physical and mental health problems. Most common are impaired lung function followed by fatigue, depression and memory impairment. In most of those affected the symptoms usually persist for at least 2 years after the initial infection and many are unable to return to work. Even cases who had mild initial disease can experience these symptoms, although those with severe disease are at higher of risk of being affected by long Covid [41, 42].

Origin of Covid-19

The origin of SARS CoV-2 has generated heated discussion. There is general agreement that the virus first emerged in Wuhan city in the Hubei province of China. The unanswered question is where it came from. There are two main theories. One holds that the virus was transmitted from an animal to a human and then spread to human to human. The alternative view is that the virus originated in a laboratory in Wuhan, where a researcher was accidently infected and then passed the infection on to other people [43].

The animal to human hypothesis is plausible because animal to human spillovers have happened frequently, not just SARS and MERS but also HIV, Ebola and the Black Death. Evidence from the early studies on Covid-19 suggested that the most likely source was the Huanan market in Wuhan city. Most of the early cases of Covid-19 occurred in central Wuhan, with the highest density of cases in the area around the market. An analysis of the first 425 cases revealed that over half (55%) were linked to the market. However, a subsequent WHO investigation found that although many of the early cases were associated with the market, there was insufficient evidence that it was the source of the outbreak. Confirmation of the animal-to-human hypothesis was not possible because the initial spillover event(s) were unlikely to be noticed or recorded [43–45].

Another theory was that the virus had leaked from a research laboratory. This hypothesis was initially dismissed as implausible by several authoritative organisations, including the World Health Organization. However, many scientists argued that the laboratory origin of the virus was possible and should be investigated further. One reason is that human pathogens have accidentally escaped many times from laboratories. Between 2000 and 2021, a total of 309 cases of laboratory leaks were identified from countries in the Americas, Europe Africa and Asia [45–47].

The laboratory leak theory is plausible because Wuhan is a major centre for research on viruses, with a remit to identify coronaviruses that might be able to cause outbreaks in humans. In 2017, researchers in Wuhan identified 11 new coronaviruses from horseshoe bats. One of these was very likely to be the immediate ancestor of the 2003 SARS virus, and three others had spike proteins that enabled them to infect human cells. The presence of this research centre in the city where the Covid-19 pandemic originated naturally gave support to the possibility that SARS CoV-2 had accidentally leaked from a laboratory [48].

Currently most scientists believe that the evidence is strongest for the animal-to-human theory, albeit it falls short of being totally convincing. A new piece of evidence provides additional support for the animal origin: the early cases in Wuhan were caused by two separate strains of the virus, labelled A and B. It is more likely that these resulted from separate animal-to-human spillover events than from two laboratory leaks. Further, there is strong evidence against the laboratory leak theory. Several studies of the genome of SARS CoV-2 have concluded that viruses cultured in a laboratory, or had been genetically manipulated, were very unlikely to have been the source of the pandemic. The methods of genetic engineering leave identifiable footprints, and none of these have been detected in the viruses spreading in community settings [46, 49, 50].

Conspiracy Theories

Covid-19 has attracted more than its fair share of conspiracy theories. An early theory in the United States was that the pandemic was a hoax intended to derail Donald Trump's 2019 re-election campaign. Bill Gates was the bogey man for two theories. One suggested that he created the virus so that he could make money by selling a vaccine. The other claimed that he was using the vaccine to implant chips in people's heads so he could monitor their behaviour. The 5G mobile network was also blamed for the spread of the virus, possibly because 5G was being rolled out when Covid-19 struck. It was also widely claimed that the nasal swab test for Covid-19 was infecting people with the virus. Genetically modified crops have been accused of causing genetic contamination, creating an environment in which the virus is more easily spread [51–53].

There are several claims that the virus was engineered as a biological weapon. One theory is that China created a virus to attack America, while another holds that the US military deliberately released it in China. It is also suggested that top business leaders, or some invisible elite, created the virus to destabilise the world order for their financial or political gain [52–54].

How the Virus Is Transmitted

SARS CoV-2 is mainly spread in the cough or sneeze of an infected person. Initially it was thought that the disease was spread by inhaling large virus-laden droplets. This theory provided the justification for two-metre physical distancing, as these droplets fall to the floor quickly. Touching the surfaces contaminated by droplets could also transmit the infection, hence the emphasis on handwashing and surface cleaning. However, as evidence accumulated, it became clear that smaller aerosol particles could also spread the virus. These aerosols stay suspended in the air for longer and are wafted about by air currents, infecting people at distances much greater than two metres. Additional measures, particularly improved ventilation of indoor spaces and the use of high-grade face masks, are needed to reduce the spread by aerosols [55, 56].

A key feature of Covid-19 is that infection mainly occurs in superspreading events, in which a few individuals spread the disease to many other people. It is not clear what factors lead to superspreading, although close contact in spaces with poor ventilation plays a role. This can happen when groups of people meet for extended periods such as travelling in a bus, attending church, singing in a choir, visiting a coffee shop or a bar. Prolonged exposure in larger gatherings, such as in aeroplanes, workplaces, business conferences, schools and hospitals, carry a higher risk multiple of exposures. Isolated environments such as nursing homes, prisons, cruise ships and naval vessels, in which people spend long periods in close proximity, are very high risk for disease transmission [57, 58].

Given that the risk of superspreading was recognised in early 2020, it is surprising that large organised events were allowed to take place. Two examples highlight the consequences. The Sturgis Motorcycle Rally in South Dakota on 7–16 August 2020 attracted almost 500,000 visitors. Although events spaces were crowded and often poorly ventilated, preventive measures such as mask wearing and physical distancing were neglected. This contributed to the spread of the infection across 17 states in the United States. Possibly the largest mass gathering is the Kumbh Mela, a Hindu religious festival that attracts tens of millions of worshippers. The main concession to Covid-19 in the April 2021 gathering was to shorten the duration of the festival from 100 days to 30 days. In crowded spaces where physical distancing was not possible, the number of new cases in India increased from 60,000 per day at the beginning of April to reach a peak of 400,000 per day by the end of the festival. Case numbers then plateaued for several days, before gradually subsiding to 150,000 by the end of May [59, 60].

Secondary Spillover and Spillback

Many animal species can be infected by contact with infected humans in what are called secondary spillover events. Humans can transfer the disease to pets such as hamsters and domestic cats and dogs. Animals in zoos are also susceptible. The first reported secondary spillover in a zoo was from animal handlers to a Malayan tiger in New York. The tiger developed a chronic cough and passed the infections to other tigers. White-tailed deer are particularly susceptible to secondary spillover from humans because their receptor for SARS CoV-2 is very similar to that of humans. Multiple spillover events have led to sustained deer-to-deer transmission. This creates the risk of spillback: transfer of the virus from animals back to humans. Several cases of spillback from these deer have been identified in the United States and Canada [61–63].

The possibility of spillback is taken seriously. Early in the Covid-19 pandemic, April 2020, humans transmitted Covid 19 to the animals in a farm that raised mink for their fur. By June it had spread widely among mink in Denmark, where there were also spillbacks to humans. It was subsequently established that the spillback virus had mutated to a form that could partially escape the immunity that humans had acquired following a first infection. To prevent any further spillback events all 17 million farmed mink in Denmark were culled [64].

Control Measures

Many types of intervention were used by governments to tackle the pandemic. Effective strategies include closing of schools, workplaces, restaurants and cinemas, international and within country travel restrictions and banning large public gatherings. Other individual-level measures, such as mask wearing and physical distancing, also reduce disease transmission. As would be expected, high levels of adherence to these restrictions were important for maximum effectiveness. Systems of test and trace, in which infected individuals are identified and all their close contacts are tested, also helped control the pandemic. All these interventions were most effective when the rates of infection were low such as in the early in the pandemic. Their impact was much less when disease transmission rates were high [65].

The combination of control measures used, and the vigour with which they were applied, varied greatly between countries. These characteristics allow policies to be broadly divided into two groups, mitigation or elimination. Although there is overlap between these groups, the essential difference between them is the aim of the policies. Mitigation was intended to have a limited impact on virus spread, whereas elimination sought to reduce infection to very low levels. Another major difference is that one preferred using voluntary regulations and the other placed emphasis on compulsory measures [66].

Mitigation

Most countries adopted a mitigation that reduced the rates of infection to what were considered acceptable levels. A common aim was to 'flatten the curve', to keep the number of cases sufficiently low so that healthcare systems could cope with the demand. Large gatherings were discouraged or cancelled, physical distancing and mask wearing were strongly encouraged as was working at home. Policies frequently changed over time. For example, the UK began with a policy of letting people become infected until the population gained herd immunity. It was only when it realised that the healthcare system would be overwhelmed by an avalanche of cases that lockdown measures were gradually imposed. Austria, Switzerland and Germany initially relied on voluntary measures such as physical distancing and working from home. As these failed to reduce infection rates sufficiently, most countries moved towards elimination strategies such as mandatory closures of borders and schools [67–69].

Elimination

The elimination strategy aimed at reducing the number of infections to close to zero. Many of the same control measures are applied but in a more aggressive manner and often for extended periods of time. Initially China only locked down Wuhan and 15 other cities in Hubei province. Then as the infection spread across the country, China implemented a dynamic zero-Covid policy of very strict border controls, lockdowns and other aggressive control measures particularly mass testing and quarantine. By 18 March 2020 it had successfully reduced infection rates to the point where only sporadic cases, interspersed with small outbreaks, continued to occur [70, 71].

Four other countries—Singapore, Hong Kong, Taiwan and Vietnam—responded rapidly to the pandemic. All were geographically close to China and had suffered from the impact of the SARS outbreaks in 2003. As a result, these countries had well-developed pandemic preparedness plans which were quickly implemented. The first actions were border controls and travel restriction, quickly followed by mask wearing, physical distancing, closures of schools and religious centres, bans on large gatherings and large-scale test and trace programmes [11, 72–75].

Evidence for the first 14 months of the pandemic showed that elimination countries had a 25-fold lower mortality than the mitigation ones. However, when sustained this strategy has serious adverse effects on peoples' physical and mental health, social well-being and education, as well as substantial economic costs because of disruptions to trade and manufacturing industries. All the countries that initially chose the elimination route gradually switched to mitigation strategies. The decisions to relax eradication policies were made much easier by the development of vaccines which substantially reduced the risk of infection and prevented serious illness and death [68, 76, 77].

The Vaccines

The rapid development of vaccines to protect against SARS CoV-2 infection was a triumph of modern science. Previously it took up to 14 years to design, develop and test a vaccine for effectiveness and then obtain regulatory approval for clinical use. But for Covid-19 it took less than a year for the first vaccine to be approved for use. This remarkable achievement was the result of two factors. Several decades of research had identified methods that both simplified the process of producing vaccines and improved their effectiveness. At the same time a detailed study of the SARS and MERS showed that the spike protein was central to the transmission of coronaviruses. Then when the Covid-19 pandemic began, funding was provided to researchers to develop vaccines that targeted the spike and the manufacturers received funding to test and mass-produce these novel vaccines [78–80].

Formal clinical trials showed that the vaccines were highly effective against symptomatic disease. Although all approved vaccines were effective, those that used the new mRNA technology provided a higher level of protection than the others. A review of the studies that evaluated the effective of the vaccines as they were used in routine immunisation programmes confirmed the high levels of protection against being infected, developing severe disease, hospitalisation and death. In the first 21 months of use, the vaccine is estimated to have prevented 152 million cases of Covid-19 and saved over 2 million lives. Further, by reducing healthcare costs and avoiding loss of economic productivity it has saved $155 billion. The effectiveness of the vaccine waned only slightly over time. At 6 months after vaccination the level protection fell by 25% but for severe disease it only reduced by 10%. Vaccination provides the best method of controlling the Covid-19 pandemic [81–83].

Vaccine Hesitancy

Despite the effectiveness and safety of the vaccines, many people are reluctant to be immunised. Some refuse outright to be vaccinated, and others have serious misgivings about it. Rates of vaccine acceptance vary around the world, but are high in most countries in the Americas and in Western Europe. Acceptance rates are lower in Eastern Europe, with Russia having a very low rate. Many countries in Africa have high rates, although others have much lower rates. Several factors contribute to reluctance to be vaccinated, particularly low levels of trust in health professionals and governments, and beliefs that the risk of infection and the severity disease are low. The most pernicious factor is the widespread dissemination of fake news, inaccurate and misleading information on social media. As the Director General of the World Health Organization commented: 'Fake news spreads faster and more easily than this virus and is just as dangerous' [84–86].

Inequitable Distribution of Vaccines

The massive efforts to develop and distribute billions of Covid-19 vaccines has been described as both 'an incredible achievement and a terrible indictment' of high-income countries. Even in the early rollout of the vaccine, the issue of vaccine nationalism, inequity of access across countries, was causing concern. The high-income countries prioritised their own populations, leaving limited supplies for low- and middle-income countries. These less well-off countries were unable to manufacture their own vaccines because ownership of intellectual property rights was held by the companies who manufactured the vaccines. Those companies were located in, and benefitted from funding provided by, the high-income countries. Low- and middle-income countries were left struggling [87, 88].

There is a compelling argument that it would be in the interests of the rich countries to donate vaccines to other countries so that all countries have high rates of immunisation. Sharing vaccines equally will reduce the risk of travel-related infections in all countries. More importantly, populations with low levels of immunity provide ideal conditions for the emergence of new variants. Hundreds of thousands of people will be infected as the virus spreads, making it more likely that rare mutations will occur. A few of these viruses could be more infectious or could cause more severe illness. This will threaten the high-income countries as much as the low- and middle-income ones. The experience of the end stage of the campaign to eradicate polio from the world is encapsulated in the phrase "polio anywhere is a risk everywhere"; it describes the challenge posed by small numbers of unvaccinated people. For Covid-19 the statement could be modified to 'low vaccination rates anywhere will spread new variants everywhere' [88–90].

New Variants

Early in the pandemic, the most common symptoms of SARS CoV-2 infection were fever, a chronic cough, loss of taste or smell, shortness of breath, fatigue and headache. As the pandemic progressed a new variant emerged which was more infectious but with a reduced severity of disease. In addition, loss of the sense of taste and smell and chronic coughing were much less common. Although the original strain of SARS -CoV2 was highly infectious, the virus keeps evolving to become even better at infecting people. New variants emerge because mutations in the spike protein make the virus more infectious. An important mutation, labelled D614G, emerged in early 2020, and by the end of that year it accounted for 95% of Covid-19 cases. By being able to infect more people more quickly, it outperformed the original strain [91–93].

There followed a series of new variants. Alpha, which was more infectious than the strain with the D614G mutation, became dominant in the early months of 2021. It was soon replaced by the Delta variant which was even more infectious and had the advantage of being good at immune escape; that is, it was less susceptible to the immunity conferred by vaccination or previous infection [34].

Omicron, which emerged in May 2022, was the most infectious variant so far. It has over 30 mutations in the spike protein which enable it to replicate much faster than the Delta variant. It also causes milder symptoms than the other variants. Several sublineages of Omicron emerged about the same time with two, BA.1 and BA.2, causing concern. BA.1 was the first to become globally dominant, but BA.2 quickly overtook it. As of February 2024, a new Omicron descendant, JN.1, was the dominant globally. It was more transmissible and was better at immune escape. Fortunately there was no reduction in vaccine effectiveness against severe disease. JN.1 now has a descendant, KP.3, that may become the new dominant variant. SARS CoV-2 just keeps generating new variants that spread across the world [34, 94, 95].

When Will It End?

On 5 May 2023 the World Health Organization (WHO) declared that Covid-19 was no longer a public health emergency of international concern. This was based on the continuing falls in the number of deaths and admissions to hospitals. The plan is that countries should move from an emergency response mode to a planned programme of long-term management. At present this is the sensible route, but it is based on the hope is that there will be no future variants that combine high infectivity, immune escape and increased severity of disease. Although there no indication that such a variant will emerge, SARS CoV-2 is remarkably adept at mutating [96–98].

As part of the transition process WHO has emphasised that the virus is still a major threat to health and encouraged countries 'to maintain sufficient capacity, operational readiness and flexibility to scale up during surges of COVID 19'. It also recognised that countries have other pressing health problems, and that they will divert facilities and staff to ensure they are making the best use of available resources. The challenge is to balance the possibility of a virulent new variant against the certainty that lives could be saved by spending money on other diseases. It is hard to escape the conclusion that certainty will win against possibility, and resources will be transferred to other priorities [97, 98].

Whatever decisions are made, Covid-19 infections will continue for years to come. One likely outcome is that SARS CoV-2 will cause illness and death at the level of outbreaks of winter flu. And, like flu, the impact will be lessened by vaccinating vulnerable people (mainly the elderly and those with serious medical conditions). An even better outcome would be if SARS CoV-2 became like the human coronaviruses that cause the common cold, with mainly mild illnesses in the winter months. That form of ending would fit well with the last line of the poem 'The Hollow Men' by T S Eliot. The original text was: 'This is the way the world ends Not with a bang but a whimper'. For Covid-19 it would be: 'this is the way the pandemic ends, not with a bang but an ongoing whimper' Let us hope that is what happens.

References

1. Murray, C. J., Lopez, A. D., Chin, B., Feehan, D., & Hill, K. H. (2006). Estimation of potential global pandemic influenza mortality on the basis of vital registry data from the 1918-20 pandemic: A quantitative analysis. *Lancet, 368*(9554), 2211–2218.
2. Bell, E., Tappero, J. W., Ijaz, K., Bartee, M., Fernandez, J., Burris, H., et al. (2017). Joint external evaluation-development and scale-up of global multisectoral health capacity evaluation process. *Emerging Infectious Diseases, 23*(13), S33–S39.
3. Sirleaf, E. J., & Clark, H. (2021). Report of the independent panel for pandemic preparedness and response: Making COVID 19 the last pandemic. *Lancet, 398*(10295), 101–103.
4. World Health Organization. (2024). WHO Covid 19 Dashboard. https://data.who.int/dashboards/covid19/cases?n=c
5. Filip, R., Gheorghita Puscaselu, R., Anchidin-Norocel, L., Dimian, M., & Savage, W. K. (2022). Global challenges to public health care systems during the COVID 19 pandemic: A review of pandemic measures and problems. *Journal of Personalized Medicine, 12*(8), 1295.
6. Worobey, M. (2021). Dissecting the early COVID 19 cases in Wuhan. *Science, 374*(6572), 1202–1204.

7. Wu, Z., & McGoogan, J. M. (2020). Characteristics of and important lessons from the coronavirus disease 2019 (COVID 19) outbreak in China: Summary of a report of 72 314 cases from the Chinese center for disease control and prevention. *Journal of the American Medical Association, 323*(13), 1239–1242.
8. Holmes, E. C., Goldstein, S. A., Rasmussen, A. L., Robertson, D. L., Crits-Christoph, A., Wertheim, J. O., et al. (2021). The origins of SARS-CoV-2: A critical review. *Cell, 184*(19), 4848–4856.
9. Wu, J. T., Leung, K., & Leung, G. M. (2020). Nowcasting and forecasting the potential domestic and international spread of the 2019-nCoV outbreak originating in Wuhan, China: A modelling study. *Lancet, 395*(10225), 689–697.
10. Zhang, Y., Zhang, A., & Wang, J. (2020). Exploring the roles of high-speed train, air and coach services in the spread of COVID 19 in China. *Transport Policy, 94*, 34–42.
11. Su, S. F., & Han, Y. Y. (2020). How Taiwan, a non-WHO member, takes actions in response to COVID 19. *Journal of Global Health, 10*(1), 010380.
12. Lau, H., Khosrawipour, V., Kocbach, P., Mikolajczyk, A., Ichii, H., Zacharski, M., et al. (2020). The association between international and domestic air traffic and the coronavirus (COVID 19) outbreak. *Journal of Microbiology, Immunology, and Infection, 53*(3), 467–472.
13. Durrheim, D. N., Gostin, L. O., & Moodley, K. (2020). When does a major outbreak become a public health emergency of international concern? *The Lancet Infectious Diseases, 20*(8), 887–889.
14. World Health Organization. (2020). Coronavirus disease 2019 (COVID 19) situation report—40. https://www.who.int/publications/m/item/situation-report%2D%2D-40
15. World Health Organization. (2020). Coronavirus disease (COVID 19) situation report—162: World Health Organization. https://www.who.int/docs/default-source/coronaviruse/20200630-Covid 9-sitrep-162.pdf?sfvrsn=e00a5466_2
16. Cucinotta, D., & Vanelli, M. (2020). WHO declares COVID 19 a pandemic. *Acta Bio-Medica, 91*(1), 157–160.
17. Chorba, T. (2020). The concept of the crown and its potential role in the downfall of coronavirus. *Emerging Infectious Diseases, 26*, 2303–2305.
18. Lin, C. N., Chan, K. R., Ooi, E. E., Chiou, M. T., Hoang, M., Hsueh, P. R., et al. (2021). Animal coronavirus diseases: Parallels with COVID 19 in humans. *Viruses, 13*(8), 1507.

19. Su, S., Wong, G., Shi, W., Liu, J., Lai, A. C. K., Zhou, J., et al. (2016). Epidemiology, genetic recombination, and pathogenesis of coronaviruses. *Trends in Microbiology, 24*(6), 490–502.
20. Hulswit, R. J., de Haan, C. A., & Bosch, B. J. (2016). Coronavirus spike protein and tropism changes. *Advances in Virus Research, 96*, 29–57.
21. Menachery, V. D., Graham, R. L., & Baric, R. S. (2017). Jumping species-a mechanism for coronavirus persistence and survival. *Current Opinion in Virology, 23*, 1–7.
22. Tang, G., Liu, Z., & Chen, D. (2022). Human coronaviruses: Origin, host and receptor. *Journal of Clinical Virology, 155*, 105246.
23. Chan-Yeung, M., & Xu, R. H. (2003). SARS: Epidemiology. *Respirology, 8*(Suppl 1), S9–S14.
24. Shi, Z., & Hu, Z. (2008). A review of studies on animal reservoirs of the SARS coronavirus. *Virus Research, 133*(1), 74–87.
25. Poutanen, S. M., & McGeer, A. J. (2004). Transmission and control of SARS. *Current Infectious Disease Reports, 6*(3), 220–227.
26. Noy, I., & Sharlan, S. (2019). *The 2003 severe acute respiratory syndrome epidemic: A retroactive examination of economic costs*. Asian Development Bank.
27. Zaki, A. M., van Boheemen, S., Bestebroer, T. M., Osterhaus, A. D., & Fouchier, R. A. (2012). Isolation of a novel coronavirus from a man with pneumonia in Saudi Arabia. *The New England Journal of Medicine, 367*(19), 1814–1820.
28. The WHO MERS-CoV Research Group. (2013). State of knowledge and data gaps of Middle East respiratory syndrome coronavirus (MERS-CoV) in humans. *PLoS Current, 12*, 5.
29. Al-Abdallat, M. M., Payne, D. C., Alqasrawi, S., Rha, B., Tohme, R. A., Abedi, G. R., et al. (2014). Hospital-associated outbreak of Middle East respiratory syndrome coronavirus: A serologic, epidemiologic, and clinical description. *Clinical Infectious Diseases, 59*(9), 1225–1233.
30. Mohd, H. A., Al-Tawfiq, J. A., & Memish, Z. A. (2016). Middle east respiratory syndrome coronavirus (MERS-CoV) origin and animal reservoir. *Virology Journal, 13*, 87.
31. Killerby, M. E., Biggs, H. M., Midgley, C. M., Gerber, S. I., & Watson, J. T. (2020). Middle east respiratory syndrome coronavirus transmission. *Emerging Infectious Diseases, 26*(2), 191–198.
32. Conzade, R., Grant, R., Malik, M. R., Elkholy, A., Elhakim, M., Samhouri, D., et al. (2018). Reported direct and indirect contact with dromedary camels among laboratory-confirmed MERS-CoV cases. *Viruses, 10*(8), 425.

33. Hui, D. S. (2016). Super-spreading events of MERS-CoV infection. *Lancet, 388*(10048), 942–943.
34. Jacobs, J. L., Haidar, G., & Mellors, J. W. (2023). COVID 19: Challenges of viral variants. *Annual Review of Medicine, 74*, 31–53.
35. World Health Organization. 2022. Middle East respiratory syndrome: Global summary and assessment of risk - 16 November 2022: World Health Organization. https://www.who.int/publications/i/item/WHO-MERS-RA-2022.1
36. Dudas, G., Carvalho, L. M., Rambaut, A., & Bedford, T. (2018). MERS-CoV spillover at the camel-human interface. *eLife, 7*, e31257.
37. Long, B., Carius, B. M., Chavez, S., Liang, S. Y., Brady, W. J., Koyfman, A., et al. (2022). Clinical update on COVID 19 for the emergency clinician: Presentation and evaluation. *The American Journal of Emergency Medicine, 54*, 46–57.
38. Struyf, T., Deeks, J., Dinnes, J., et al. (2022). Signs and symptoms to determine if a patient presenting in primary care or hospital outpatient settings has COVID 19. *Cochrane Database of Systematic Reviews, 5*(5), CD013665.
39. Cevik, M., Kuppalli, K., Kindrachuk, J., & Peiris, M. (2020). Virology, transmission, and pathogenesis of SARS-CoV-2. *BMJ, 371*, m3862.
40. Wolff, D., Nee, S., Hickey, N. S., & Marschollek, M. (2021). Risk factors for Covid 19 severity and fatality: A structured literature review. *Infection, 49*(1), 15–28.
41. Zeng, N., Zhao, Y. M., Yan, W., Li, C., Lu, Q. D., Liu, L., et al. (2023). A systematic review and meta-analysis of long term physical and mental sequelae of COVID 19 pandemic: Call for research priority and action. *Molecular Psychiatry, 28*(1), 423–433.
42. Rahmati, M., Udeh, R., Yon, D. K., Lee, S. W., Dolja-Gore, X., Mc, E. M., et al. (2023). A systematic review and meta-analysis of long-term sequelae of COVID 19 2-year after SARS-CoV-2 infection: A call to action for neurological, physical, and psychological sciences. *Journal of Medical Virology, 95*(6), e28852.
43. Alwine, J. C., Casadevall, A., Enquist, L. W., Goodrum, F. D., & Imperiale, M. J. (2023). A critical analysis of the evidence for the SARS-CoV-2 origin hypotheses. *Journal of Virology, 8*, e0036523.
44. Worobey, M., Levy, J. I., Malpica Serrano, L., Crits-Christoph, A., Pekar, J. E., Goldstein, S. A., et al. (2022). The huanan seafood wholesale market in Wuhan was the early epicenter of the COVID 19 pandemic. *Science, 377*(6609), 951–959.

45. Joint WHO-China Study Team Report. (2021). WHO-convened global study of origins of SARS-CoV-2: China Part.
46. Bahry, D. (2023). Rational discourse on virology and pandemics. *MBio, 14*, e0031323.
47. Blacksell, S. D., Dhawan, S., Kusumoto, M., Le, K. K., Summermatter, K., O'Keefe, J., et al. (2024). Laboratory-acquired infections and pathogen escapes worldwide between 2000 and 2021: A scoping review. *Lancet Microbe, 5*(2), e194–e202.
48. Hu, B., Zeng, L. P., Yang, X. L., Ge, X. Y., Zhang, W., Li, B., et al. (2017). Discovery of a rich gene pool of bat SARS-related coronaviruses provides new insights into the origin of SARS coronavirus. *PLoS Pathogens, 13*(11), e1006698.
49. Pekar, J. E., Magee, A., Parker, E., Moshiri, N., Izhikevich, K., Havens, J. L., et al. (2022). The molecular epidemiology of multiple zoonotic origins of SARS-CoV-2. *Science, 377*(6609), 960–966.
50. Goodrum, F., Lowen, A. C., Lakdawala, S., Alwine, J., Casadevall, A., Imperiale, M. J., et al. (2023). Virology under the microscope-a call for rational discourse. *mSphere, 8*(2), e0003423.
51. Stein, R. A., Ometa, O., Pachtman Shetty, S., Katz, A., Popitiu, M. I., & Brotherton, R. (2021). Conspiracy theories in the era of COVID 19: A tale of two pandemics. *International Journal of Clinical Practice, 75*(2), e13778.
52. Tsamakis, K., Tsiptsios, D., Stubbs, B., Ma, R., Romano, E., Mueller, C., et al. (2022). Summarising data and factors associated with COVID 19 related conspiracy theories in the first year of the pandemic: A systematic review and narrative synthesis. *BMC Psychology, 10*(1), 244.
53. Lynas M.. (2021); Covid: Top 10 current conspiracy theories 2020. https://allianceforscience.cornell.edu/blog/2020/04/covid-top-10-current-conspiracy-theories/
54. Ghebreyesus T. (2020); Munich security conference: World Health Organization. https://www.who.int/director-general/speeches/detail/munich-security-conference
55. de Crane, D.' H. S., Parisi, G., Lisson, M., Bruyère, O., Donneau, A. F., Fontaine, S., et al. (2023). Systematic review of the key factors influencing the indoor airborne spread of SARS-CoV-2. *Pathogens, 12*(3), 382.
56. Duval, D., Palmer, J. C., Tudge, I., Pearce-Smith, N., O'Connell, E., Bennett, A., et al. (2022). Long distance airborne transmission of SARS-CoV-2: rapid systematic review. *BMJ, 377*, e068743.

57. Meyerowitz, E. A., Richterman, A., Gandhi, R. T., & Sax, P. E. (2021). Transmission of SARS-CoV-2: A review of viral, host, and environmental factors. *Annals of Internal Medicine, 174*(1), 69–79.
58. Lakdawala, S. S., & Menachery, V. D. (2021). Catch me if you can: Superspreading of COVID 19. *Trends in Microbiology, 29*(10), 919–929.
59. Carter, R. J., Rose, D. A., Sabo, R. T., Clayton, J., Steinberg, J., & Anderson, M. (2021). Widespread severe acute respiratory syndrome coronavirus 2 transmission among attendees at a large motorcycle rally and their contacts, 30 US jurisdictions, august-September, 2020. *Clinical Infectious Diseases, 73*(Suppl 1), S106–S109.
60. Rocha, I. C. N., Pelayo, M. G. A., & Rackimuthu, S. (2021). Kumbh Mela religious gathering as a massive superspreading event: Potential culprit for the exponential surge of COVID 19 cases in India. *The American Journal of Tropical Medicine and Hygiene, 105*(4), 868–871.
61. Sparrer, M. N., Hodges, N. F., Sherman, T., VandeWoude, S., Bosco-Lauth, A. M., & Mayo, C. E. (2023). Role of spillover and spillback in SARS-CoV-2 transmission and the importance of one health in understanding the dynamics of the COVID 19 pandemic. *Journal of Clinical Microbiology, 61*, e0161022.
62. Feng, A., Bevins, S., Chandler, J., DeLiberto, T. J., Ghai, R., Lantz, K., et al. (2023). Transmission of SARS-CoV-2 in free-ranging white-tailed deer in the United States. *Nature Communications, 14*(1), 4078.
63. Pickering, B., Lung, O., Maguire, F., Kruczkiewicz, P., Kotwa, J. D., Buchanan, T., et al. (2022). Divergent SARS-CoV-2 variant emerges in white-tailed deer with deer-to-human transmission. *Nature Microbiology, 7*(12), 2011–2024.
64. Tan, C. C. S., Lam, S. D., Richard, D., Owen, C. J., Berchtold, D., Orengo, C., et al. (2022). Transmission of SARS-CoV-2 from humans to animals and potential host adaptation. *Nature Communications, 13*(1), 2988.
65. Walport, M., Ashton, J., Barclay, W., et al. (2023). *COVID 19: examining the effectiveness of non-pharmaceutical interventions*. The Royal Society. https://royalsociety.org/-/media/policy/projects/impact-non-pharmaceutical-interventions-on-Covid19-transmission/
66. Wu, S., Neill, R., De Foo, C., Chua, A. Q., Jung, A. S., Haldane, V., et al. (2021). Aggressive containment, suppression, and mitigation of Covid 19: Lessons learnt from eight countries. *BMJ, 375*, e067508.

67. Lu, G., Razum, O., Jahn, A., Zhang, Y., Sutton, B., Sridhar, D., et al. (2021). COVID 19 in Germany and China: Mitigation versus elimination strategy. *Global Health Action, 14*(1), 1875601.
68. Ye, H., Tang, Y., Zhou, Z., et al. (2023). The trade-off between economic development and pandemic control: Strategy identification and effect analysis. *Journal of Development Effectiveness, 16*, 187–205.
69. Daud, A. (2022). Five common misconceptions regarding flattening-the-curve of COVID 19. *History and Philosophy of Life Sciences, 44*, 41–47.
70. Zhao, Z., Zhou, Y., Li, W., Fan, X., Huang, Q., Tang, Z., et al. (2022). Discussion on China's anti-epidemic response based on the protocol on prevention and control of coronavirus disease 2019 from Chinese authority. *International Journal of Health Planning and Management, 37*(3), 1205–1220.
71. Liu, M., Shi, L., Chen, H., Wang, X., Yang, M., Jiao, J., et al. (2022). Comparison between China and Brazil in the two waves of COVID 19 prevention and control. *Journal of Epidemiology and Global Health, 12*(2), 168–181.
72. Cowling, B. J., Ali, S. T., Ng, T. W. Y., Tsang, T. K., Li, J. C. M., Fong, M. W., et al. (2020). Impact assessment of non-pharmaceutical interventions against coronavirus disease 2019 and influenza in Hong Kong: An observational study. *The Lancet Public Health, 5*(5), e279–e288.
73. Oh, J., Lee, J. K., Schwarz, D., Ratcliffe, H. L., Markuns, J. F., & Hirschhorn, L. R. (2020). National response to COVID 19 in the Republic of Korea and lessons learned for other countries. *Health System Reform, 6*(1), e1753464.
74. Van Tan, L. (2021). COVID 19 control in Vietnam. *Nature Immunology, 22*(3), 261.
75. Lee, W. C., & Ong, C. Y. (2020). Overview of rapid mitigating strategies in Singapore during the COVID 19 pandemic. *Public Health, 185*, 15–17.
76. Oliu-Barton, M., Pradelski, B. S. R., Algan, Y., Baker, M. G., Binagwaho, A., Dore, G. J., et al. (2022). Elimination versus mitigation of SARS-CoV-2 in the presence of effective vaccines. *The Lancet Global Health, 10*(1), e142–e147.
77. Adams, S., Lancaster, K., & Rhodes, T. (2023). Undoing elimination: Modelling Australia's way out of the COVID 19 pandemic. *Global Public Health, 18*(1), 2195899.
78. Mao, W., Zimmerman, A., Urli Hodges, E., Ortiz, E., Dods, G., Taylor, A., et al. (2023). Comparing research and development, launch, and scale up timelines of 18 vaccines: Lessons learnt from COVID 19 and implications for other infectious diseases. *BMJ Global Health, 8*(9), e012855.

79. Saleh, A., Qamar, S., Tekin, A., et al. (2021). Vaccine development throughout history. *Cureus, 13*(7), e16635.
80. Ball, P. (2021). The lightning-fast quest for COVID vaccines - and what it means for other diseases. *Nature, 589*(7840), 16–18.
81. Zheng, C., Shao, W., Chen, X., Zhang, B., Wang, G., & Zhang, W. (2022). Real-world effectiveness of COVID 19 vaccines: A literature review and meta-analysis. *International Journal of Infectious Diseases, 114*, 252–260.
82. Yang, J., Vaghela, S., Yarnoff, B., De Boisvilliers, S., Di Fusco, M., Wiemken, T. L., et al. (2023). Estimated global public health and economic impact of COVID 19 vaccines in the pre-omicron era using real-world empirical data. *Expert Review of Vaccines, 22*(1), 54–65.
83. Feikin, D. R., Higdon, M. M., Abu-Raddad, L. J., Andrews, N., Araos, R., Goldberg, Y., et al. (2022). Duration of effectiveness of vaccines against SARS-CoV-2 infection and COVID 19 disease: results of a systematic review and meta-regression. *Lancet, 399*(10328), 924–944.
84. Sallam, M., Al-Sanafi, M., & Sallam, M. (2022). A global map of COVID 19 vaccine acceptance rates per country: An updated concise narrative review. *Journal of Multidisciplinary Healthcare, 15*, 21–45.
85. Pires, C. (2022). Global predictors of COVID 19 vaccine hesitancy: A systematic review. *Vaccines (Basel), 10*(8), 1349.
86. Islam, M. S., Kamal, A. M., Kabir, A., Southern, D. L., Khan, S. H., Hasan, S. M. M., et al. (2021). COVID 19 vaccine rumors and conspiracy theories: The need for cognitive inoculation against misinformation to improve vaccine adherence. *PLoS One, 16*(5), e0251605.
87. Riaz, M. M. A., Ahmad, U., Mohan, A., Dos Santos Costa, A. C., Khan, H., Babar, M. S., et al. (2021). Global impact of vaccine nationalism during COVID 19 pandemic. *Tropical Medicine and Health, 49*(1), 101.
88. Farlow, A., Torreele, E., Gray, G., Ruxrungtham, K., Rees, H., Prasad, S., et al. (2023). The future of epidemic and pandemic vaccines to serve global public health needs. *Vaccines (Basel), 11*(3), 690.
89. Moore, S., Hill, E. M., Dyson, L., Tildesley, M. J., & Keeling, M. J. (2022). Retrospectively modeling the effects of increased global vaccine sharing on the COVID 19 pandemic. *Nature Medicine, 28*(11), 2416–2423.
90. Shivam, S., Weitz, J. S., & Wardi, Y. (2022). Vaccine stockpile sharing for selfish objectives. *PLOS Global Public Health, 2*(12), e0001312.
91. Fan, Y., Li, X., Zhang, L., Wan, S., Zhang, L., & Zhou, F. (2022). SARS-CoV-2 omicron variant: Recent progress and future perspectives. *Signal Transduction and Targeted Therapy, 7*(1), 141.

92. Isabel, S., Graña-Miraglia, L., Gutierrez, J. M., Bundalovic-Torma, C., Groves, H. E., Isabel, M. R., et al. (2020). Evolutionary and structural analyses of SARS-CoV-2 D614G spike protein mutation now documented worldwide. *Scientific Reports, 10*(1), 14031.
93. Magazine, N., Zhang, T., Wu, Y., McGee, M. C., Veggiani, G., & Huang, W. (2022). Mutations and evolution of the SARS-CoV-2 spike protein. *Viruses, 14*(3), 640.
94. Esper, F. P., Adhikari, T. M., Tu, Z. J., Cheng, Y. W., El-Haddad, K., Farkas, D. H., et al. (2023). Alpha to omicron: Disease severity and clinical outcomes of major SARS-CoV-2 variants. *The Journal of Infectious Diseases, 227*(3), 344–352.
95. Aden, D., & Zaheer, S. (2024). Investigating the FLiRT variants of COVID 19: Is it an emerging concern? *Pathology, Research and Practice, 262*, 155542.
96. Wise, J. (2023). Covid 19: WHO declares end of global health emergency. *BMJ, 381*, 1041.
97. World Health Organization. (2023). *From emergency response to long-term Covid 19 disease management: sustaining gains made during the Covid 19 pandemic*. World Health Organization.
98. World Health Organization. (2024). *COVID 19 epidemiological update—17 September 2024*. World Health Organization.

Summing up: How Pandemics Begin, Spread Globally and End

Pandemics share three features. They are almost always unexpected, suddenly emerging in one place then spreading around the world. As well as causing serious illness and death, pandemics are also responsible for a great deal of social disruption and substantial economic loss. Finally, governments are usually unprepared to deal with pandemics. The recent Covid-19 pandemic is testimony to the confusion and blunders that characterised the responses in many countries. Other than these commonalities, pandemics differ in almost all their main characteristics, particularly where they come from, why they spread and how they end (if they do end) [1, 2].

Where they Come from

The origins of some pandemics are simply not known. Polio (a virus) may have been infecting humans for at least 6000 years, but the place and date of its emergence is obscure. Similarly, there are many historical references to a disease that resembles leprosy (a bacterium), but little is known about where it came from. The source of syphilis (a bacterium) has been the subject of

© The Author(s), under exclusive license to Springer Nature Singapore Pte Ltd. 2025

I. K Crombie, *Major Pandemics*, https://doi.org/10.1007/978-981-95-2081-7_14

much heated debate, but there is no convincing evidence about where it began. More is known about the other pandemics.

Some of the bacterial pathogens, such as the *Vibrio cholerae*, came directly from the physical environment (soil and water). The distant ancestors of *M. tuberculosis* also lived in the soil, but the origin of the bacterium that causes TB is unclear. Possibly it came from the soil, but it could also have jumped from an infected animal to humans. *Yersinia pestis*, the bacterium that caused the Black Death lived in the soil but had to migrate through rodents and fleas before it could infect humans.

Many viral pathogens have jumped from animals into humans. Thus, measles probably spilled over from domesticated cows, although it could have come from other animals such as goats, camels or pigs. Smallpox most likely came from animals such as camels or gerbils. The main strain of the HIV virus came from a chimpanzee. Yellow fever also spilled over from non-human primates, but it had to use a mosquito as an intermediary to transmit the virus to humans. The influenza virus can be transferred directly from aquatic birds such as gulls, geese and terns into humans, although it sometimes passes through pigs or chickens before infecting people. The source of Covid-19 is uncertain. It may have come directly from a bat but could also have infected humans through an intermediary animal in a Wuhan market. Or it may have been extracted from a bat and grown in a laboratory from where it infected humans.

The pandemics of the last 700 years have had diverse origins, but that may be changing. All the pandemics of the last 150 years have been caused by viruses that spilled over from animals. Further, over the past 70 years all the large disease outbreaks that almost became pandemics have been caused by viruses that jumped from animals to humans. One reason is that animals such as bats, rodents and non-human primates are host to a wide range of viruses and have transmitted many of them to humans. Several other animals, particularly ungulates (cloven-hoofed animals such as cows and pigs) and birds, can also transmit viruses to humans. It is a reasonable guess that the next pandemic will be caused by a virus that jumps from an animal to a human. The problem is no one knows when this will happen, nor which animal it will come from. What is likely is that human activities will increase the risk of a new pandemic [3–5].

The Increased Risk from Human Activities

Cutting down virgin forests to create land for cultivation and settlement often results in the fragmentation of forests. The once large forests are being broken into small parcels of woodland which are often surrounded by farms and houses. This greatly increases the risk of human exposure to viruses in wild animals. For example, the major Ebola outbreak in 2013 is thought to have been caused by forest fragmentation [6, 7].

The global trade in wildlife, both legal and illegal, has been likened to a gateway for new infectious diseases. It includes trading in exotic pets and the selling of ivory, rhino horn and animal furs. This trade involves about two million animals each year. Estimates put the financial value at about $23 billion. As the animals are passed between traders and then into the homes and gardens of customers, there are opportunities for new pathogens to infect humans [8, 9].

Another route for human exposure is the butchering of wild animals for human consumption. In many rural areas this is out of necessity, with the poorest households reliant on bushmeat to survive. About 150 million households consume wild animals to supplement their diets. By killing these animals and butchering them for their meat for them, people can be infected with new pathogens.

Finally there is the increasing consumption of exotic food for pleasure. In the live animal markets that provide these delicacies, animals from many species are crowded together in unsanitary conditions where they can share infectious diseases. The major epidemic of SARS (severe acute respiratory syndrome) almost certainly sprang from a palm civet (a mongoose-like animal) that was sold in an exotic food market in Guangdong Province in southern China. These markets provide an ongoing risk of novel infectious diseases in humans [10–12].

Why they Spread

To become a pandemic, an infectious disease needs to be quickly spread among people in a local area, then expand to other areas and finally around the world. Several methods are available. The respiratory route is a common method of person to person spread. Flu, measles, leprosy, smallpox, tuberculosis and Covid-19 are all spread this way. When humans gather in poorly ventilated spaces, the risk of inhaling the droplets and aerosols produced by the coughs and sneezes of an infected individual is high. Overcrowding increases the spread of infectious diseases because people 'talk, laugh, eat, cough, sneeze and sleep close together' [13].

Sexual intercourse has been a highly successful method for spreading syphilis and HIV. It benefits from the popularity of sex. The risk of infection increases with the frequency of intercourse and the number of partners. Not using a condom and anal intercourse are particularly high-risk activities.

Another method is transmission by biting insects. They were responsible for the Black Death (fleas) and for yellow fever (mosquitoes). The geographical range of mosquitoes restricts the spread of yellow fever to tropical and subtropical regions. Fleas are not subject to the same limitation, but with increased attention to personal hygiene in the modern era, this method of spread is unlikely to be successful.

Pandemics of cholera and polio were spread by consumption of contaminated water and foodstuffs. This method of transmission is referred to as the oral/faecal route because after being swallowed the pathogen is excreted, contaminating the local environment. Poor personal hygiene and limited access to sanitation facilities are central to the proliferation of these diseases. It is unlikely that a future pandemic will be spread in this way because so many countries have high-quality sanitary facilities.

Modern Civilisation and the Spread of Pandemics

When a new pandemic emerges three facets of modern civilisation will greatly assist its spread: global travel, climate change and urbanisation. The extent and the speed of spread of a pandemic depend on the means of transport available. The Black Death was mainly carried by traders on horse-back or in wagons, so it was restricted to the Eurasia and North Africa. But with the developments of ocean-going ships, the new pandemics of smallpox and syphilis could be spread globally in a matter of months. Other transport innovations, steamships and railways, reduced the time for the long-distance travel of the Spanish flu pandemic to several days. Whereas the very rapid spread of Covid-19 benefitted from air travel which could transport the infection around the world in less than 24 hours.

Global warming could also increase the geographical range of the mosquito, bringing many tropical diseases to regions which currently have temperate climates. These include unpleasant infections such as West Nile fever, Dengue fever, Zika fever, Chikungunya break bone fever and Japanese encephalitis. All these diseases are caused by RNA viruses which could mutate to become better adapted to mosquito and more infectious and severe in humans. Any of them could cause a global pandemic [14–16].

When people lived in small communities and seldom travelled far, infectious diseases would have limited spread. But with urbanisation, they gather in large communities and have social networks that range for beyond of people that live nearby. This provides ideal conditions for the spread of diseases. Pathogens that are spread by the respiratory route and by sexual intercourse will flourish in such environments. For the past 70 years there has been a mass movement of people from rural to urban areas. In 1950 only 30% of people lived in urban areas. This increased to 54% in 2014 and it is predicted to reach 66% by 2050. By that time the global population will be about 10 billion people. Any new highly infectious disease will thrive in these vast conglomerations of people [17, 18].

How they End

Most pandemics do not end. The one exception is smallpox, a disease which was eradicated by mass vaccination. Polio is on the verge of a similar fate and has been for the last 25 years. But the emergence of virus strains that are resistant to vaccines together with insufficient funding, local armed conflicts and vaccine hesitancy has prevented the eradication of this virus.

Measles was also identified as suitable for eradication, as there is a very effective vaccine and no animal reservoirs to seed new outbreaks. The measles vaccination programme suffers from many of the challenges that afflict polio (insufficient funding, local armed conflicts and vaccine hesitancy). But it has the additional problem of a disease which is so highly infectious that in populations with lowish levels of immunity even a single case will quickly lead to a large outbreak. As measles is still highly active, with about 200,000 deaths each year, eradication is a distant prospect.

The Black Death, or more correctly the plague, ended after almost 500 years of infecting people. It most likely disappeared because of the combined effects of quarantine, improved building techniques and climate change. However, during the third plague pandemic the bacterium *Yersinia pestis* established reservoirs of infection around the world. These continue to seed small disease outbreaks. Rather than having ended, the plague has been marginalised and is unlikely to cause another pandemic.

Pandemic cholera gradually faded away, as improved sanitation and provision of clean drinking water diminished the opportunities for disease transmission. However, small outbreaks will continue to emerge. The third cholera pandemic created environmental reservoirs from which new infections are seeded. These are amplified by poverty and poor quality sanitation. It seems certain that there will be new outbreaks of cholera for many years to come.

Yellow fever is another disease that is sustained by environmental reservoirs, the tropical rainforests in Africa and South America. They frequently seed new outbreaks that are quickly spread by the human adapted mosquito *Aedes aegypti*. Forest fragmentation plays an important role in increasing the chances that humans will be infected. As vaccination of all people that live near the tropical rainforests is probably unfeasible, yellow fever outbreaks seem destined to continue [19, 20].

Leprosy is still causing untold thousands of cases of disfigurement and disability each year. The combination of a moderately effective vaccine and a highly effective treatment has substantially reduced the burden of infection. Initially the fall in the number of new cases was rapid, but much less progress has been made in the last few years. With increased effort and additional funding, the number of new cases could be greatly reduced, but the end of leprosy is likely to be in the distant future.

Some pathogens mutate to cause less severe symptoms. This was the fate of the pandemics of flu, and Covid-19 may also follow this route. But there is little evidence that other pandemics will fade away because of reduced virulence. Three current pandemics, tuberculosis (TB), syphilis and HIV, show no signs of fading away. TB became a major killer over 300 years ago and currently causes over 1 million deaths each year. The infection is most common in low and middle income countries, where poverty, undernutrition, HIV and drug resistance sustain its spread. With more effective vaccines, better diagnostic tests and new drug treatments, and a reduction in poverty, TB infection may finally be controlled.

Controlling syphilis and HIV is challenging because they are mainly spread by sexual intercourse. Admittedly HIV has only been causing widespread disease for about 40 years, but the fact that syphilis is still a major problem after 500 years suggests that there are deep-seated reasons that make sexually transmitted diseases difficult to control. The combination of the popularity of sex as a leisure pursuit, an apparent reluctance of some people to adopt safe sex practices and the difficulties governments face in reducing high-risk practices impedes efforts to reduce disease transmission.

The Next Pandemic

Given the frequency of pandemics over the last few hundred years, it seems more than likely that a new pandemic will occur in the near future. Although there is a general consensus on this, no one knows when it will happen or what the disease will be. A new flu pandemic is an ever-present risk, but there are many other pathogens that could become pandemic. Concern about this led the World Health Organization (WHO) to create a list of priority diseases. It was based on two criteria: they should have the potential to spread widely, causing severe illness and death. They are also diseases for which there are no effective drugs or vaccines.

From an initial long list of 28 diseases, 10 were identified as high priority: Ebola and Marburg, Zika, SARS, MERS, Nipah and Hendra, Lassa fever, River Valley fever and Crimean-Congo haemorrhagic fever. They are all RNA viruses, which means they could mutate rapidly to become better at infecting humans. WHO's aim was to stimulate research into novel diagnostic tests, treatments and vaccines. If this is successful, the world would be better prepared to tackle the next pandemic [21–23].

Because it is not possible to predict the cause of the next pandemic, WHO created a special category 'Disease X'. It was intended to raise awareness that the next pandemic could begin with a few cases of an atypical new infectious disease. In doing so, WHO demonstrated considerable foresight. Only 2 years after disease X was announced, the world was gripped by Covid-19 [24].

An independent research group has also evaluated the risk of spillover of viruses from animals to humans. Their top 50 viruses included most of those in the WHO priority list. Among the other viruses rated as high risk were several that are well known (rabies, simian foamy virus and hepatitis E virus). Some others with high scores are less familiar (Seoul virus, Bombali virus and Laguna Negra virus). It seems there is no shortage of candidates for a new pandemic [25].

There is also a strong possibility that the next pandemic will be a previously unknown virus. The last two human pandemics, HIV/AIDS and Covid-19, were novel viruses and both resulted from animal to human spillovers. Certainly, there are many viral species that could jump into humans. Between 1930 and 2018 a total of 6571 viruses of mammals had been identified, and researchers are actively seeking new ones. It is estimated that there are about 1.7 million undiscovered viruses that could infect humans [26, 27].

Pandemics and Preparedness

Pandemics are incredibly destructive. Millions of people die, and substantial healthcare costs are incurred in treating the sick and developing and distributing new vaccines and treatments. Economic productivity can also fall because industrial supply chains are disrupted. To minimise the impact of a new pandemic several global organisations have produced detailed preparedness strategies. The United Nations General Assembly has recently published its Political Declaration on Preparedness. These findings have been incorporated in the World Health Organization's Pandemic Agreement. A final draft of this document was released in 2024. In addition, the World Bank has created a fund to support essential activities for pandemic preparedness. Although there have been criticisms, particularly about equity of vaccine sharing, substantial progress has been made in negotiating international support for these proposals [28–30].

A complementary approach, and one which receives less attention from the global organisations, is to identify viruses with pandemic potential before they spillover from animals into humans. Scientists are currently developing predictive tools to screen for such viruses. By studying a virus's characteristics and the environment in which it lives, measures could be put in place to reduce the risk of it emerging to cause a pandemic. This strategy does have weaknesses. There are concerns that the rate of virus discovery far exceeds the capacity to conduct in-depth assessments of pandemic potential. It is also difficult to control the drivers of viral emergence, such as preventing deforestation and reducing the global wildlife trade. Although promising, the value of this approach may not be realised in the near future [27, 31, 32].

But there is a compelling reason to be fully prepared for the next pandemic: the worst-case scenario. A novel respiratory RNA virus could cause a devastating pandemic if it contained several features that maximise the spread of infection. These are:

- Infection causes coughing and sneezing and generates virus-laden aerosols.
- These aerosols remain infectious for many hours.
- The virus particles in the aerosols are highly infectious.
- Infection causes many asymptomatic cases who can spread the disease for several weeks.
- The virus seriously impairs the human immune system.
- Symptomatic disease results in severe illness and has a high mortality rate.
- The virus mutates rapidly so that it quickly becomes resistant to vaccines.

This hypothetical virus combines properties from SARS-CoV-2, measles and HIV, so it is biologically plausible that a worst-case virus could exist. With high volumes of international travel and an increasingly urbanised population, it would spread like wildfire. The loss of life and the accompanying social and economic disruption could be far greater than from previous pandemics. Let us hope that such a virus does not emerge from an animal. Or, if it did, that there was a high state of pandemic preparedness.

Possibly the main threat is complacency. As several years pass with no sign of a new pandemic, governments may mothball their plans and divert resources to more urgent concerns. The lessons of Covid-19 could be forgotten and preparedness would be a distant memory.

Postscript November 2025

This review of pandemics has shown how global efforts, together with substantial funding, have greatly reduced suffering and death from many serious diseases. In addition, there are increasing efforts to detect and control newly emergent diseases, particularly those that might cause future pandemics. But with the election of Donald Trump as president of the USA in November 2024, all of that has changed.

The United States had a proud record of being the major contributor to global health through its financial support to WHO, and for the prevention and control of a host of diseases. But, starting in early 2025, funding for WHO and a wide range of health programmes including HIV, TB, malaria, polio, measles and diphtheria has been severely cut back or completely withdrawn. Even maternal and child health has not escaped this fate. Not only will existing targets for disease prevention be missed, there is likely to be a sustained increase in disease frequency and death. The low- and middle-income countries will be most affected. However, if the phrase 'an outbreak anywhere is a threat everywhere' has any substance to it, then the US may also suffer. With the rise in diseases such as HIV and syphilis, Americans travelling overseas will be at an increased risk. Tourists and business people visiting the US may inadvertently spread these diseases among the local population [33–35].

The United States has the right to withdraw from funding global health programmes. But it seems unfortunate that the views of one president are at variance with those of most presidents over the last 50 years. The massive cuts in global health funding will squander the benefits of past investments. They will also seriously degrade the monitoring of new infectious outbreaks and impair the ability to quickly contain any such outbreaks. Potential future pandemics will thrive more readily when global disease control efforts have been eroded. Donald Trump may be remembered as the president who made the world a more perilous place [33–35].

References

1. Gaskell, J., Stoker, G., Jennings, W., et al. (2020). Covid-19 and the blunders of our governments: Long-run system failings aggravated by political choices. *The Political Quarterly, 91*(3), 523–533.
2. Mellish, T., Luzmore, N., & Shahbaz, A. (2020). Why were the UK and USA unprepared for the COVID-19 pandemic? The systemic weaknesses of neoliberalism: A comparison between the UK, USA, Germany, and South Korea. *Journal of Global Faultlines, 7*(1), 9–45.
3. Jones, K. E., Patel, N. G., Levy, M. A., Storeygard, A., Balk, D., Gittleman, J. L., et al. (2008). Global trends in emerging infectious diseases. *Nature, 451*(7181), 990–993.
4. Bernstein, A. S., Ando, A. W., Loch-Temzelides, T., Vale, M. M., Li, B. V., Li, H., et al. (2022). The costs and benefits of primary prevention of zoonotic pandemics. *Science Advances, 8*(5), eabl4183.
5. Mollentze, N., & Streicker, D. G. (2020). Viral zoonotic risk is homogenous among taxonomic orders of mammalian and avian reservoir hosts. *Proceedings of the National Academy of Sciences of the United States of America, 117*(17), 9423–9430.
6. Daszak, P., Amuasi, J., das Neves, C., et al. (2020). *IPBES workshop on biodiversity and pandemics.* IPBES Secretariat.
7. Rulli, M. C., Santini, M., Hayman, D. T., & D'Odorico, P. (2017). The nexus between forest fragmentation in Africa and Ebola virus disease outbreaks. *Scientific Reports, 7,* 41613.
8. Bezerra-Santos, M. A., Mendoza-Roldan, J. A., Thompson, R. C. A., Dantas-Torres, F., & Otranto, D. (2021). Illegal wildlife trade: A gateway to zoonotic infectious diseases. *Trends in Parasitology, 37*(3), 181–184.

9. Can, Ö. E., D'Cruze, N., & Macdonald, D. W. (2019). Dealing in deadly pathogens: Taking stock of the legal trade in live wildlife and potential risks to human health. *Global Ecology and Conservation, 17*, e00515.
10. Nielsen, M., Meilby, H., Smith-Hall, C., et al. (2018). The importance of wild meat in the global south. *Ecological Economics, 146*, 696–705.
11. Naguib, M. M., Li, R., Ling, J., Grace, D., Nguyen-Viet, H., & Lindahl, J. F. (2021). Live and wet markets: Food access versus the risk of disease emergence. *Trends in Microbiology, 29*(7), 573–581.
12. Galindo-González, J. (2022). Live animal markets: Identifying the origins of emerging infectious diseases. *Current Opinion in Environmental Science & Health, 25*, 100310.
13. McNicholas, A., Lennon, D., Crampton, P., & Howden-Chapman, P. (2000). Overcrowding and infectious diseases--when will we learn the lessons of our past? *The New Zealand Medical Journal, 113*(1121), 453–454.
14. Wu, X., Lu, Y., Zhou, S., Chen, L., & Xu, B. (2016). Impact of climate change on human infectious diseases: Empirical evidence and human adaptation. *Environment International, 86*, 14–23.
15. Rocklöv, J., & Dubrow, R. (2020). Climate change: An enduring challenge for vector-borne disease prevention and control. *Nature Immunology, 21*(5), 479–483.
16. Yu, X., & Cheng, G. (2022). Adaptive evolution as a driving force of the emergence and re-emergence of mosquito-borne viral diseases. *Viruses, 14*(2), 435.
17. Kii, M. (2021). Projecting future populations of urban agglomerations around the world and through the 21st century. *npj Urban Sustainability, 1*, 10.
18. Leeson, G. (2018). The growth, ageing and urbanisation of our world. *Journal of Population Ageing, 11*, 107–115.
19. Ajayi, A., & Smith, S. I. (2019). Recurrent cholera epidemics in Africa: Which way forward? A literature review. *Infection, 47*(3), 341–349.
20. Islam, M. S., Zaman, M. H., Islam, M. S., Ahmed, N., & Clemens, J. D. (2020). Environmental reservoirs of vibrio cholerae. *Vaccine, 38*(Suppl 1), A52–a62.
21. Bloom, D. E., & Cadarette, D. (2019). Infectious disease threats in the twenty-first century: Strengthening the global response. *Frontiers in Immunology, 10*, 549.
22. Mehand, M. S., Al-Shorbaji, F., Millett, P., & Murgue, B. (2018). The WHO R&D blueprint: 2018 review of emerging infectious diseases requiring urgent research and development efforts. *Antiviral Research, 159*, 63–67.

23. Jonkmans, N., D'Acremont, V., & Flahault, A. (2021). Scoping future outbreaks: A scoping review on the outbreak prediction of the WHO blueprint list of priority diseases. *BMJ Global Health, 6*(9), e006623.
24. van Doorn, H. R. (2021). The epidemiology of emerging infectious diseases and pandemics. *Medicine (Abingdon), 49*(10), 659–662.
25. Grange, Z. L., Goldstein, T., Johnson, C. K., Anthony, S., Gilardi, K., Daszak, P., et al. (2021). Ranking the risk of animal-to-human spillover for newly discovered viruses. *Proceedings of the National Academy of Sciences of the United States of America, 118*(15), e2002324118.
26. Gibb, R., Albery, G. F., Mollentze, N., Eskew, E. A., Brierley, L., Ryan, S. J., et al. (2022). Mammal virus diversity estimates are unstable due to accelerating discovery effort. *Biology Letters, 18*(1), 20210427.
27. Lawrence, P., Heung, M., Nave, J., Henkel, C., & Escudero-Pérez, B. (2023). The natural virome and pandemic potential: Disease X. *Current Opinion in Virology, 63*, 101377.
28. Grabar-Kitarović, K., & Phumaphi, J. (2023). A crisis of trust in pandemic prevention, preparedness, and response. *Lancet, 402*(10414), 1730–1732.
29. Lancet, T. (2024). The pandemic treaty: Shameful and unjust. *Lancet, 403*(10429), 781.
30. Boyce, M. R., Sorrell, E. M., & Standley, C. J. (2023). An early analysis of the World Bank's pandemic fund: A new fund for pandemic prevention, preparedness and response. *BMJ Global Health, 8*(1), e011172.
31. Albery, G. F., Becker, D. J., Brierley, L., Brook, C. E., Christofferson, R. C., Cohen, L. E., et al. (2021). The science of the host-virus network. *Nature Microbiology, 6*(12), 1483–1492.
32. Mollentze, N., & Streicker, D. G. (2023). Predicting zoonotic potential of viruses: Where are we? *Current Opinion in Virology, 61*, 101346.
33. Aremu S. O., Adamu, A. I., Obeta, O. K., et al. (2025). The United States withdrawal from the world health organization (WHO), its implications for global health governance. *Globalization and Health, 21*, 48. https://doi.org/10.1186/s12992-025-01137-0
34. Poddar, A., & Rao, S. R. (2025). The consequences of US retreat from the global health security leadership. *Health Security, 23*(4), 282–288. https://doi.org/10.1089/hs.2025.0055
35. Desai, A. N., Jacobs, E., Ogedegbe, O., et al. (2025). The global public health imperative—Where do we go from here? *JAMA Network Open, 8*(5), e2517283. https://doi.org/10.1001/jamanetworkopen.2025.17283

Glossary

Endemic, Epidemic and Pandemic

Endemic

Endemic diseases are those which occur regularly in a country, community or area. In this context, regularly means that cases of a disease occur in most years.

Epidemic

An epidemic is an increase in the frequency of a disease in a country of region. It often occurs suddenly and produces a large number of new cases of the disease.

Pandemic

A pandemic is an epidemic that has spread across several countries. Many pandemics have some additional features such as: rapid spread, affecting large numbers of people or causing severe illness.

© The Author(s), under exclusive license to Springer Nature Singapore Pte Ltd. 2025

I. K Crombie, *Major Pandemics*, https://doi.org/10.1007/978-981-95-2081-7

RNA

Some viruses have RNA as their genetic information instead of DNA. RNA is similar to DNA except that thymine (T) is replaced by a molecule called uracil (U). So RNA viruses code their information using sequences of A,U,C and G.

Genes

Genetic material, whether RNA of DNA, is organised into sections called genes. These contain the information to make specific proteins. Some proteins form the building block of cells, others help repair cells, promote growth in children or protect against invading pathogens. In short, proteins make life possible.

Mutations

A mutation is a change (error) in the sequence of the molecules in a piece of DNA or RNA. For example, when an A is replaced by a G, or even when the A is simply missed out. Mutations can change the way a molecule functions in an organism, usually to make it work less well, but occasionally to improve its function. Very rarely organisms such as a bacterium or a virus will acquire a series of mutations that enable them to thrive. As a result they will multiply more quickly their neighbours.

Pathogens

A pathogen is any organism that causes disease in an animal, plant or bacterium. This book focuses on two types of pathogen: bacteria and viruses.

Bacteria

A bacterium is a small single-celled organism encased in a hard shell. Most bacteria can survive on their own, but some can also invade animals and grow in them. Many bacteria live happily in humans, helping to promote good health. However, pathogenic bacteria can cause serious illness.

Viruses

Viruses are very small and simple organisms, comprising a piece of genetic material wrapped up in a protein coat. They need to invade cells to replicate, using specific receptors (see below) to do so. Once inside they hijack the cells' biochemistry to make multiple copies of the genetic material and the proteins for the coat. Viruses are essentially parasites, although sometimes they can help their host by killing off invading bacteria.

There are millions upon millions of different viruses. The human gut alone contains over 140,000 different viral species. The origin of viruses remains a bit of a mystery. They may have evolved independently of cells and bacteria, or they may be degraded versions of cells or parts of cells.

Retroviruses

Most viruses store their genetic information in DNA. Retroviruses use RNA. They can convert the RNA into DNA which can then be incorporated into the DNA of the host cell. This enables them to make lots of new viruses.

Receptors

Viruses have special molecules on their surface that can bind to other molecules (receptors) on the surface of cells. The process is analogous to a key and a lock; only one type of virus molecule can bind to a specific receptor. The process of binding enables the virus to enter the cell.

Species

Species is the term given to a group in which all the individuals are very similar. The word 'genus' is used to identify several species which are broadly similar. For example the genus Mycobacteria includes the bacteria which cause tuberculosis (*Mycobacterium tuberculosis*) and those of leprosy (*Mycobacterium leprae*). All organisms are identified by their genus and species names.

Spillover

A spillover occurs when a pathogen is transmitted from one animal species to another one in which it can successfully replicate. The term is commonly used for the transfer from animals to humans.

Spillback

Spillback is often called reverse spillover. The pathogen is transferred from human to an animal, usually to a different species from the one involved in the initial spillover.

Zoonosis

A zoonosis is an infection that is transmitted from animals to humans.

Measuring Infectiousness

The Basic Reproduction Number R_0

R_0 is the average number of new cases of a disease caused the individuals who are currently infected. Measles is often reported to have an R_0 of about 12–18, which means that on average each infected person transmits the disease to another 12–18 people. In fact, estimates of R_0 vary substantially across the studies which try to measure infectiousness. For measles they range from 3.7 to 200 depending on study quality, the measurement techniques used and the characteristics of the population measured (e.g. population density, patterns of social mixing and birth rate). R_0 is not just a measure of a pathogen's infectivity; it also depends on human behaviour and social organisation.

Herd Immunity

Herd immunity is the proportion of a population who are immune to a disease. If the proportion is high, an infection can only spread slowly. When lots of people are immune then most infected individuals will be unlikely to encounter people who are susceptible, so will be unable to transmit the disease. The threshold for herd immunity depends on the infectiousness of a disease, R_0, in a particular setting. Using commonly accepted values measles is highly infectious with an R_0 of 12–18, so has a threshold of 83–94%. In contrast, mumps has an R_0 of about 5 and a threshold of about 80%. However, these thresholds may be unreliable given the potential variability in R_0.

The Immune System

Humans, like all animals, have evolved two methods of identifying and destroying pathogens.

Innate Immunity

The innate immune system is the first to respond. It releases a fixed, but large, variety of proteins and cells. These come from a library of defences that is genetically programmed, based on the experiences of pathogens that attacked our far distant ancestors. It is a blind shotgun approach in which only a few of the proteins and cells can identify, attack and kill the invading pathogen. However, the system quickly mass-produces the ones that are effective. It also alerts the adaptive immune system that the body is under threat.

Adaptive Immunity

The adaptive immune system is slower to respond, but it targets specific locations on the surface of the pathogen. One way it does this is to produce antibodies. These are proteins which attach to specific regions of the pathogen surface and help neutralise it. The other method uses certain types of cell that recognise and kill foreign pathogens. The immune system remembers which pathogens have invaded previously. If infected again the system mounts a much faster targetted attack.

Vaccination

Vaccination is a method of priming the body's immune system so that it responds quickly when invaded by a new pathogen. Each vaccine is specific to one pathogen.

Vaccine Hesitancy

Vaccine hesitancy is the reluctance to be vaccinated because of fears that the vaccine is harmful or ineffective.

Dating of Disease Outbreaks

The abbreviations BCE (Before Common Era) and CE (Common Era) are preferred to the abbreviations BC (Before Christ) and AD (Anno Domini, the year of Christ's birth). They are used to achieve religious neutrality but convey the same information. Thus, 520 BCE is equivalent to 520 BC, and 290 CE to 290 AD.

Contagious and Infectious

Contagious

A contagious disease is one that is spread from person to person. The term derives from the Latin *contigere*, meaning to touch. Originally contagious was restricted to diseases which were spread by physical contact, for example glandular fever (the kissing disease). More recently the definition has expanded to include any form of human to human spread, such as inhaling tiny infectious particles from the breath of a person with influenza.

Infectious

Infectious diseases are those that are spread by any means such as by contaminated water (cholera), by insects (mosquitoes and malaria) or by or injecting drugs with a syringe that is contaminated with HIV. This term includes all of the diseases that are contagious.

Genetic Material: DNA, RNA and Mutations

DNA

DNA stores the genetic information of all animals, plants, bacteria and many viruses. It provides a set of instructions on how to make the molecules that living organisms need to grow and survive. The information is coded in specific sequences of four molecules labelled A,T,C and G (short for adenine, thymine, cytosine and guanine).

FSC
www.fsc.org
MIX
Papier | Fördert gute Waldnutzung
FSC® C083411

Kolibri 360 GmbH
Ferdinand-Jühlke-Straße 7
99095 Erfurt, Deutschland
produktsicherheit@kolibri360.de